Fertility and ART
in Medical Disorders

Fertility and ART in Medical Disorders

Editors

Harpreet Kaur
MBBS MD DNB MRCOG (UK) Fellowship Reproductive Medicine (FNB)
Associate Professor
Department of Obstetrics and Gynecology
All India Institute of Medical Sciences
Bilaspur, Himachal Pradesh, India

Sweta Gupta
MD MRCOG (Lon) MSc (Reproduction and Development, UK)
FRCOG (Lon) Fellowship Reproductive Medicine and ART (Lon)
Director, IVF
Max Healthcare Ltd
New Delhi/Noida, India

Foreword
Kanad Dev Nayar

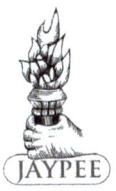

JAYPEE BROTHERS MEDICAL PUBLISHERS
The Health Sciences Publisher
New Delhi | London

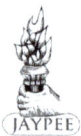 **Jaypee Brothers Medical Publishers (P) Ltd**

Headquarters

Jaypee Brothers Medical Publishers (P) Ltd
EMCA House, 23/23-B
Ansari Road, Daryaganj
New Delhi 110 002, India
Landline: +91-11-23272143, +91-11-23272703
+91-11-23282021, +91-11-23245672
Email: jaypee@jaypeebrothers.com

Corporate Office

Jaypee Brothers Medical Publishers (P) Ltd
4838/24, Ansari Road, Daryaganj
New Delhi 110 002, India
Phone: +91-11-43574357
Fax: +91-11-43574314
Email: jaypee@jaypeebrothers.com

Overseas Office

JP Medical Ltd
83 Victoria Street, London
SW1H 0HW (UK)
Phone: +44 20 3170 8910
Fax: +44 (0)20 3008 6180
Email: info@jpmedpub.com

Website: www.jaypeebrothers.com
Website: www.jaypeedigital.com

© 2024, Jaypee Brothers Medical Publishers

The views and opinions expressed in this book are solely those of the original contributor(s)/author(s) and do not necessarily represent those of editor(s) or publisher of the book.

All rights reserved. No part of this publication may be reproduced, stored or transmitted in any form or by any means, electronic, mechanical, photocopying, recording or otherwise, without the prior permission in writing of the publishers.

All brand names and product names used in this book are trade names, service marks, trademarks or registered trademarks of their respective owners. The publisher is not associated with any product or vendor mentioned in this book.

Medical knowledge and practice change constantly. This book is designed to provide accurate, authoritative information about the subject matter in question. However, readers are advised to check the most current information available on procedures included and check information from the manufacturer of each product to be administered, to verify the recommended dose, formula, method and duration of administration, adverse effects and contraindications. It is the responsibility of the practitioner to take all appropriate safety precautions. Neither the publisher nor the author(s)/editor(s) assume any liability for any injury and/or damage to persons or property arising from or related to use of material in this book.

This book is sold on the understanding that the publisher is not engaged in providing professional medical services. If such advice or services are required, the services of a competent medical professional should be sought.

Every effort has been made where necessary to contact holders of copyright to obtain permission to reproduce copyright material. If any have been inadvertently overlooked, the publisher will be pleased to make the necessary arrangements at the first opportunity.

Inquiries for bulk sales may be solicited at: jaypee@jaypeebrothers.com

Fertility and ART in Medical Disorders

First Edition: **2024**

ISBN: 978-93-5696-312-2

Dedicated to
All our patients

Contributors

Ankita Sethi
MD DNB MRCOG DM Reproductive Medicine
Consultant
Akanksha IVF Centre
New Delhi, India

Arpita Ray MD MRCOG
Honorary Professor
New Vision University, Georgia, USA
Consultant and Lead Clinician
Bourn Hall Fertility Clinic, UK

Ashis Bassi
MBBS MPhil MD FRCP
Honorary Senior Lecturer
University of Liverpool
Consultant Gastroenterologist
Associate Medical Director
St Helens and Knowsley Hospitals
Liverpool, UK

Atri Pal
MCh (Reproductive Medicine & Surgery)
Consultant Fertility Specialist and
Fertility Enhancing Surgeon
Renew Healthcare
Kolkata, West Bengal, India

Bharti Jain
DNB (Radiology)
Director
KJIVF and Laparoscopy Centre
New Delhi/Faridabad, India

Bharti Joshi MD
Assistant Professor
Department of Obstetrics and
Gynecology
Postgraduate Institute of Medical
Education and Research
Chandigarh, India

Fiona Dennison
MBChB MRCOG
Consultant Obstetrician, Specialist in
Maternal Medicine
Ayrshire Maternity Hospital
NHS Ayrshire and Arran Health Board,
Scotland

Garima Patel DM
Resident (Reproductive Medicine)
Department of Obstetrics and
Gynecology
All India Institute of Medical Sciences
New Delhi, India

Harpreet Kaur
MBBS MD DNB MRCOG (UK) Fellowship
Reproductive Medicine (FNB)
Associate Professor
Department of Obstetrics and
Gynecology
All India Institute of Medical Sciences
Bilaspur, Himachal Pradesh, India

Kanad Dev Nayar
MD DGO Dip Obst (Ireland) FICOG
Chief Consultant and Head
(Infertility & IVF)
Akanksha IVF Centre
Mata Chanan Devi Hospital
New Delhi, India
President, Indian Fertility Society
(2022–24)

KN Singh
MBBS MD DNB (Nephro) FISN FISOT
Senior Consultant
Department of Nephrology and
Multiorgan Transplant
Indraprastha Apollo Hospital
New Delhi, India

Contributors

Kuldeep Jain MD FART (Singapore)
Director
KJIVF and Laparoscopy Centre
New Delhi/Faridabad, India

Maansi Jain
MS (Obs & Gyne) Diploma Clinical ART
Fellowship Reproductive Medicine and
Surgery, Singapore
Consultant and Laparoscopic Surgeon
KJIVF and Laparoscopy Center
New Delhi, India

Naila Mohiuddin MD
Research Scholar
Medical Health and Research Institute
Hyderabad, Telangana, India

Neeta Singh MBBS MD
Professor (Reproductive Medicine)
Department of Obstetrics and
Gynecology
All India Institute of Medical Sciences
New Delhi, India

(Col) Pankaj Talwar VSM
Fertility and Embryology Consultant
CEO and Director
i-Ceat (Clinical and Embryology
Academy of ART)
i-HOMaa Fertility Clinics
i-Consult (IVF & IUI Consultancy
Services) Global Virtual Library
New Delhi, India

Pikee Saxena MD
Director Professor
Department of Obstetrics and
Gynecology
Lady Hardinge Medical College and SSKH
New Delhi, India

Preyander Singh Thakur
MBBS MD (Medicine) DM (Endocrinology &
Metabolism)
Associate Professor
Endocrinology and Metabolism
All India Institute of Medical Sciences
Bilaspur, Himachal Pradesh, India

Priyank Kothari
MBBS MS MCh (Uro) DNB (Genitourinary
Surgery)
Consultant Uro-Andrologist
Assistant Professor
Department of Urology
Dr BYL Nair Charitable Hospital
Mumbai, Maharashtra, India

Puja Kumari
MBBS MS (Obs & Gyne)
Senior Consultant
Crysta IVF
Patna, Bihar, India

Rajesh Vijayvergiya
MD DM FSCAI FACC FISES FESC
Professor
Department of Cardiology
Postgraduate Institute of Medical
Education and Research
Chandigarh, India

Roya Rozati MD
Professor and Head
Department of Obstetrics and
Gynecology
Shadan Institute of Medical Sciences
Director
Medical Health and Research Institute
Hyderabad, Telangana, India

Rupali Goyal
MBBS DNB Dip in USG MNAMS
Senior Consultant
Apollo Assisted Reproduction Unit
Department of Obstetrics and
Gynecology
Indraprastha Apollo Hospitals
New Delhi, India

Sakshi Miglani MS
Fellow in ART
Akanksha IVF Centre
New Delhi, India

Contributors

Santanu Acharya
MBBS MD FICOG MSc FRCOG
Honorary Clinical Associate Professor
University of Glasgow
Person Responsible, Ayrshire Fertility Unit
Consultant Gynecologist and Obstetrician
University Hospital
Crosshouse, UK

Saumya Prasad
MD MS (Obstetrics & Gynecology)
Consultant
Matritava Advanced IVF and Training Center
New Delhi, India

Shahida Naghma MD
Associate Consultant
Birla Fertility and IVF
New Delhi, India

Shrinkhala Gupta MD
Fellow
Matritava Advanced IVF and Training Center
New Delhi, India

Shubhda Gupta MD
Fellow
Matritava Advanced IVF and Training Center
New Delhi, India

Smriti RC Bhatta
MBBS MD FRCOG FHEA
Senior Lecturer (Scholarship)
Deputy Lead Assessment
University of Aberdeen
Senior Clinician, Aberdeen Fertility Centre
NHS Grampian Health Board, Scotland

Sudha Prasad MD
Director
Matritava Advanced IVF and Training Center
New Delhi, India

Sujoy Dasgupta MS DNB MRCOG MSc
Consultant
Reproductive Medicine
Genome Fertility Centre
Kolkata, West Bengal, India

Surveen Ghumman Sindhu
MD (Obs & Gyne) FICOG FICMCH
Senior Director and Head
Department of IVF and Reproductive Medicine
MAX Superspecialty Hospitals
New Delhi/Gurugram, India
Professor
School of Health Sciences
Ansal University
Gurugram, Haryana, India

Sweta Gupta
MD MRCOG (Lon) MSc (Reproduction and Development, UK) FRCOG (Lon) Fellowship in Reproductive Medicine and ART (Lon)
Director, IVF
Max Healthcare Ltd
New Delhi/Noida, India

Varun Dhir MD DM
Associate Professor
Department of Rheumatology
Postgraduate Institute of Medical Education and Research
Chandigarh, India

Vidhi Chaudhary MD
Professor
Department of Obstetrics and Gynecology
Lady Hardinge Medical College and SSKH
New Delhi, India

Vilvapathy Senguttuvan Karthikeyan
MBBS MS MCh (Uro) MRCS FECSM
Microsurgical Andrologist and Urologist
Andrology Unit
Department of Urology
Apollo Hospitals
Chennai, Tamil Nadu, India

Contributors

Vineet Malhotra
MBBS MS DNB (Genitourinary Surgery)
Senior Consultant, Urologist and Andrologist
Director, VNA Hospital
New Delhi, India

Wajeeda Tabasum MD
Research Scholar
Medical Health and Research Institute
Hyderabad, Telangana, India

Foreword

I am honored and delighted to provide a foreword for the book, *Fertility and ART in Medical Disorders*. This incredible piece of literature delves into the intricate world of assisted reproductive techniques and their applications in patients with medical diseases.

In recent years, advancements in the field of reproductive medicine have revolutionized the possibilities for individuals and couples facing various medical conditions. The introduction of in-vitro fertilization (IVF) has opened doors to hope and parenthood for those who previously believed their dreams of starting a family were out of reach. This book comprehensively explores the intersection of IVF and medical diseases, shedding light on the potential solutions and challenges that arise.

The authors of this book have meticulously compiled a wealth of knowledge and expertise, drawing upon their vast experiences in reproductive medicine. Their insights into the intricacies of IVF in the setting of medical diseases are invaluable for medical professionals, researchers, and individuals navigating fertility challenges. Their meticulous attention to detail, coupled with their compassionate approach to patient care, shines through in each chapter of this book.

I have no doubt that *Fertility and ART in Medical Disorders* will serve as an invaluable resource for healthcare professionals, researchers, and clinicians who endeavor to provide the best care possible for individuals with medical diseases facing fertility challenges. This book not only broadens our knowledge but also inspires hope and fosters a deeper appreciation for the incredible advancements in assisted reproductive technologies.

I extend my heartfelt congratulations to the authors on their remarkable achievement and extend my gratitude for their dedication to advancing the field of reproductive medicine. May this book be a guiding light for those seeking answers, support, and solutions in the realm of fertility and medical diseases.

Kanad Dev Nayar
MD DGO Dip Obst (Ireland) FICOG
Chief Consultant and Head
(Infertility & IVF)
Akanksha IVF Centre
Mata Chanan Devi Hospital
New Delhi, India
President, Indian Fertility Society (2022-24)

Preface

Subfertility is prevalent in about 10–15% of reproductive age group couples. With the advancement in the technique of ART, many couples are able to conceive and fulfil their dream of parenthood which was otherwise difficult. Treatment of couples with various medical disorders is even more challenging to both the treating physician and the couple themselves. This book provides a comprehensive guide to treatment of fertility and ART in many such couples. The chapters are contributed by the authors who have expertise in the field of Reproductive Medicine and aided by multidisciplinary input from the specialists dealing with the concerned medical problems. This book will be a guide to the medical students, nurses, general physicians, specialists and researchers who are dealing with fertility and ART in the presence of medical conditions that needs meticulous attention and individualized management planning.

Harpreet Kaur
Sweta Gupta

Contents

1. **Introduction** 1
   Sweta Gupta, Harpreet Kaur

2. **Fertility and Assisted Reproductive Technology Renal Transplant** 2
   KN Singh, Rupali Goyal

3. **Assisted Reproductive Technology in Postliver Transplant** 10
   Vidhi Chaudhary, Pikee Saxena

4. **Male Fertility and Solid Organ Transplants** 20
   Vineet Malhotra, Vilvapathy Senguttuvan Karthikeyan, Priyank Kothari

5. **Fertility and Assisted Reproductive Technology in Cancer Survivors: Breast Cancer** 32
   Kanad Dev Nayar, Ankita Sethi, Sakshi Miglani

6. **Fertility and Assisted Reproductive Technology in Cancer Survivors: Endometrial Cancer** 46
   Surveen Ghumman Sindhu

7. **Fertility and Assisted Reproductive Technology in Cancer Survivors: Hereditary Cancers** 54
   Roya Rozati, Wajeeda Tabasum, Naila Mohiuddin

8. **Fertility and Assisted Reproductive Technology in Cancer Survivors: Lymphoma/Leukemia** 61
   Pankaj Talwar, Shahida Naghma

9. **Male Fertility and Cancers** 72
   Kuldeep Jain, Bharti Jain, Maansi Jain

10. **Fertility and Assisted Reproductive Technology in Obesity and Postbariatric Surgery** 82
    Sudha Prasad, Shrinkhala Gupta, Saumya Prasad, Shubhda Gupta

11. **Fertility and Assisted Reproductive Technology in Autoimmune Disorders** 92
    Bharti Joshi, Varun Dhir

12. **Fertility and Assisted Reproductive Technology in Women on Anticoagulants** 99
    Arpita Ray

13. **Fertility and Assisted Reproductive Technology in Cardiac Disease** 107
    Harpreet Kaur, Rajesh Vijayvergiya

14. **Fertility and Assisted Reproductive Technology in Chronic Renal Disease** 115
    Neeta Singh, Garima Patel

15. **Fertility and Assisted Reproductive Technology in Liver Disorders** 131
    Smriti RC Bhatta, Santanu Acharya, Fiona Dennison, Ashis Bassi

16. **Fertility and Assisted Reproductive Technology in Hypertensive Disorders** 146
    Atri Pal, Sujoy Dasgupta

17. **Fertility and Assisted Reproductive Technology in Diabetes Mellitus** 157
    Sweta Gupta, Puja Kumari, Preyander Singh Thakur

Index *169*

Chapter 1

Introduction

Sweta Gupta, Harpreet Kaur

Infertility is the inability to conceive after a year of unprotected intercourse. The incidence of subfertility has significantly increased in the last decade due to changes in the lifestyle, late marriage, sexually transmitted diseases, pollution, and medical disorders, which together have a complex effect on fertility. It has a significant negative effect on the couple psychologically, socially leading to emotional distress, anxiety, low esteem, and depression.

There had been significant advances in the field of ART in the last decade. More than five million children have been born globally through ART until now giving joy of parenthood to disheartened couples. With advancement in technology, there is a need to have guidance. Women with medical disorders such as endocrine problems (diabetes/thyroid), heart disease, coagulation disorder, renal disease, and women post-transplant undergoing fertility treatment have also increased in recent years. With advancement in diagnosis and treatment of these medical problems, nowadays, significantly more and more women can survive adulthood and plan pregnancy. Management of fertility in the presence of an underlying medical problem is a major challenge to the treating clinicians. It may require multidisciplinary input of a physician and fertility specialist and an individualized treatment approach. Almost all of them need a thorough preconceptional counseling highlighting the effect of a chronic medical condition on fertility, treatment options available and their success rate, need for multidisciplinary care, and obstetric outcome.

This book will serve as a comprehensive guide for the optimal fertility treatment to the reproductive medicine clinicians dealing with cases of infertility in the setting of medical disorders. All the chapters have been contributed by consultants experienced in fertility management with input from the concerned specialty. Every attempt has been made to present a clear management approach to women with medical disorders seeking fertility care.

Fertility and Assisted Reproductive Technology Renal Transplant

KN Singh, Rupali Goyal

■ INTRODUCTION

End-stage renal disease (ESRD) is known to be associated with fertility issues, in both males and females. The incidence may vary from as much as 30 to 90%.[1] Renal transplant is known to reverse most of these scenarios associated with reproductive function. A return of fertility occurs within 6 months to 1 year post-transplant.[2]

The first pregnancy in a post-transplant was reported 65 years back in 1958; ever since, a multitude of babies have been born following spontaneous conception.

Babies born by medically assisted reproduction (MAR) are very few. The largest case series from Turkey has reported 11 clinical pregnancies following in vitro fertilization (IVF) in 13 women, and 6 of them carried and delivered till term.[3]

Apart from the age of the patient, the extent of fertility issues would usually vary with the stage of the disease.[4]

These patients not only suffer with infertility but have a higher incidence of sexual dysfunction as well. These symptoms are usually associated with endocrinological, psychological, drugs, and vasomotor alterations in the milieu.[5]

■ ETIOPATHOGENESIS OF INFERTILITY IN POST-TRANSPLANT PATIENTS

There are multifactorial etiological factors causing fertility issues in as high as 50% of the patients.

The degree of sexual dysfunction and infertility would be dependent on various factors:
- The etiological factor responsible for causing ESRD may also affect the ovarian and testicular function, especially in chronic conditions such as diabetes and hypertensive disorders. In patients with polycystic kidney disease, which is an autosomal dominant condition, there is an association with asthenozoospermia. Patients with prune belly syndrome present with undescended testicles and infertility.

- The age of the couple presenting with infertility is one of the most important prognostic factors when it comes to treatment procedures offered. ESRD occurs in chronic conditions, so the age of either of the partners seeking fertility treatments is usually >35 years.
- Intraoperatively, during a transplant surgery in males, there is a risk of damage to the spermatic cord structures, for example, vas deferens, and a hampered testicular blood supply causing increased chances of fertility issues in the couple.[6]
- *Hormonal disturbances:* Various hormonal aberrations have been noted in post-transplant recipients—they may range from mild elevation in the pituitary gonadotropin hormones, which self-correct 3–12 months post-transplant, to persistently high levels denoting organ failure.
  Wang et al. in 2010 compared the levels of gonadotropic hormones such as luteinizing hormone (LH), follicle-stimulating hormone (FSH), prolactin pretransplant versus 4 months post-transplant. He observed that the levels were significantly higher in the pretransplant phase, which led to lower levels of testosterone and estrogen in males and females, respectively.[7]
- These patients present with a hypergonadotropic hypogonadism picture. There is an elevation in the pituitary gonadotropic hormones leading to a regulatory fall in the estrogen and testosterone levels in females and males, respectively. This presents with the features of sexual dysfunction observed in the patients with chronic kidney disease.
- *Drugs:* Patients with ESRD are usually on various drugs; apart from immunosuppressants, they might also be on drugs which lead to gonadal dysfunction, for example, antihypertensives, thiazides, aldosterone receptor blockers, and beta-adrenergic receptor blockers.
- During the renal transplant recipients, there is a small but definitive risk of injury to the vas, resulting in impaired spermatogenesis, lower semen volume, and reduced sperm motility and viability.
- In patients with postrenal transplant status, there are multiple psychological factors that further increase both sexual function and infertility among these patients.

CLINICAL PRESENTATION

Patients with renal transplant would present sexual dysfunction as well as infertility. Erectile dysfunction is a common feature, which is likely to improve only in one-half to one-fourth of the patients post-transplant. Both male and female patients present with loss of libido and also difficulty achieving orgasm.

Low levels of circulating estrogen cause females to present with excessive vaginal dryness.

Female patients usually present with an oligomenorrhea or amenorrhea during the ESRD phase. Of all women on dialysis, >90% have an irregular or absent menstrual cycle.

■ EFFECT OF TRANSPLANT ON PREGNANCY

The first ever pregnancy following a renal transplant in a recipient has been reported as early as 1958.[8]

There is paucity of data on the pregnancy outcomes in patients with pregnancy outcomes in postrenal transplant status.

A recent systematic review and meta-analysis showed that 6,712 pregnancies occurred in 4,174 kidney transplant recipients. The mean maternal age was 29.6 ± 2.4 years. The live-birth rate was 72.9%, induced abortions 12.4% [95% confidence interval (CI), 10.4–14.7], miscarriages 15.4% (95% CI, 13.8–17.2), stillbirths 5.1% (95% CI, 4.0–6.5), ectopic pregnancies 2.4% (95% CI, 1.5–3.7), preeclampsia 21.5% (95% CI, 18.5–24.9), gestational diabetes 5.7% (95% CI, 3.7–8.9), pregnancy-induced hypertension 24.1% (95% CI, 18.1–31.5), cesarean section 62.6 (95% CI 57.6–67.3), and preterm delivery 43.1% (95% CI, 38.7–47.6). The mean gestational age was 34.9 weeks, and the mean birth weight was 2,470 g.[9,10]

■ EFFECT OF PREGNANCY ON A POST-TRANSPLANT RECIPIENT

Post-transplant recipients during pregnancy are at high risks for the following:
- Graft dysfunction or rejection
- Need for dialysis during pregnancy due to rising renal parameters
- Renal transplant patients would be on immunosuppressants such as cyclosporine or tacrolimus and low-dose steroids. The blood levels of these drugs are measured every biweekly to maintain permissible levels.[11]
- Both these drugs are in category C [United States Food and Drug Administration (USFDA)] for safety in pregnancy usage although tacrolimus is known to cross the placenta, the levels in a fetus are approximately 71% of that of maternal blood concentrations. The lower fetal blood concentrations are likely due to active efflux transport of tacrolimus from the fetus toward the mother by placental P-glycoprotein. Although there are no reports of congenital malformations following use in the first trimester, cases with reversible neonatal hyperkalemia and renal impairment have been reported.[12]

■ FETAL EFFECTS OF TRANSPLANT ON PREGNANCY

There are various gamut of factors influencing the outcomes of pregnancy in renal transplant recipients.

The patients who have a higher incidence of complications during pregnancy have a higher incidence of first-trimester abortions and threatened miscarriage and are further associated with growth retardation in the latter stages of pregnancy.

These patients tend to develop early onset preeclampsia with varying degrees of proteinuria.

There is a higher incidence of associated gestational diabetes mellitus during pregnancy.

The transplant recipient patients have a higher risk of developing anemia, which would necessitate blood transfusion.

A total of 30% of these patients may develop impaired renal function, which might be mild in up to 30% of cases due to graft rejection.

In the third trimester, the patients have a higher incidence of preterm delivery and premature rupture of membranes leading to a higher incidence of admission to the neonatal intensive care unit (ICU).

The serum levels of cyclosporine or tacrolimus were measured every 2 weeks to adjust the maintenance dose.

Apart from a significantly increased incidence of preeclampsia, the transplant recipients with a history of chronic hypertension also showed a significantly higher incidence of superimposed preeclampsia.

There was an associated higher risk of operative preterm delivery by cesarean section in such patients.

■ COUNSELING IN RENAL TRANSPLANT PATIENTS

The patients who have had renal transplants, are advised to wait for a minimum period of 1 year before trying for a spontaneous conception. In 2018, the Italian Society of Nephrology, with their Kidney and Pregnancy Study group, released a best practice position statement in postrenal transplant recipient pregnancies, higher incidence of adverse maternal-fetal outcomes in patients undergoing assisted reproduction, post-transplant.[13,14]

Patients planning for motherhood do have options for pregnancy during dialysis or post-transplant stage. Patients should also be counseled for the availability of MAR techniques and their side effects. Options of surrogacy and adoption should also be discussed based on the age, profile or comorbidities, and general status of the patient.[15]

■ IMMUNOSUPPRESSION DURING PREGNANCY

The transplant patients are usually on immunosuppressive drugs for a prolonged period of time. Fetal safety concerns and risk of teratogenicity should always be discussed with the couple planning to go for motherhood.

Along with a nephrologist, the dosage of the medications needs to be adjusted to the minimum safety levels. More commonly, these patients are on corticosteroids, calcineurin inhibitors, azathioprine, and mycophenolate.

Among these drugs, the first three are considered safe with no or minimal risk of teratogenicity, whereas mycophenolate is contraindicated during pregnancy due to the higher incidence of associated teratogenicity and spontaneous abortions. Patients who are strictly on mycophenolate are advised to stop it for a minimum 6 weeks of gestation, so the risk of teratogenicity is similar to nontransplant recipients.

Corticosteroids, usually given in the form of low-dose prednisolone, have a lower concentration in fetal blood as compared to the maternal levels.

Calcineurin inhibitors, such as tacrolimus, are commonly used immunosuppressive agents and are relatively safe in pregnancy. Although no teratogenic effects have been shown in these patients, the levels need to be monitored every 2 weeks in these patients.[15,16]

■ PREGNANCY AND GRAFT FUNCTION

Apart from being an immunomodulatory state, there is an altered renal profile during pregnancy. An increase in the glomerular filtration rate is observed during pregnancy. The value of serum creatinine decreases in the first and second trimesters of pregnancy. The value rises to the prepregnancy values in the third trimester of gestation.

Studies have reported variable reports on the status of risk of graft rejection.

A recent meta-analysis demonstrated that acute rejection rates were similar in pregnant and nonpregnant recipients of transplants.

One of the most important factors responsible for the graft survival postpregnancy is dependent on the status of the prepregnancy graft function.[14,15]

■ FETAL OUTCOMES IN POST-TRANSPLANT RECIPIENTS

The fetal risks during pregnancy are not only due to the prepregnancy compromised renal function but also due to the immunosuppressive drugs administered during pregnancy.

Mycophenolate is known to cause brain dysfunction in the neonates if administered during the first trimester.

The risk of early pregnancy loss, small for gestational age fetus, and preterm delivery is more in patients with elevated serum creatinine during pregnancy. The outcomes of babies are similar in the natural conception or the MAR group.[17]

The incidence of stillbirths and early perinatal deaths within 24 hours of birth was significantly higher among the transplant group as compared to the general population.[18]

MEDICALLY ASSISTED REPRODUCTION IN TRANSPLANT PATIENTS

The first IVF pregnancy in a renal transplant recipient was reported by Lockwood et al. in 1995.[19] A long agonist protocol was followed and a double-embryo transfer resulted in a twin pregnancy. The patient delivered at 29 weeks' gestation following preterm premature rupture of membranes.[10]

In Turkey, Yaprak et al. performed a retrospective analysis of 13 patients undergoing a total of 24 IVF cycles. Among the 13 patients, 1 patient had a renal shut down; subsequently, 3 more had a 30% increase in the renal function parameters.[3]

Subsequently, there have been many cases of MAR in these patients.

The basic algorithm for management of a renal recipient stays similar to a normal infertile couple. The type of management offered to the patients would be based on the infertility indications and current graft status. The overall aim of management would be a healthy singleton live baby.

The most commonly used drugs in infertility management are clomiphene citrate, letrozole, and gonadotropins. Although there is paucity of data on the safety profile of these drugs, letrozole might be preferred over others for its antiestrogenic effects. However, the safety profile of the drugs needs to be assured before putting them to use.

High levels of estrogenic hormones can lead to hypercoagulability and thrombus formation, so the levels need to be monitored and antithrombotic prophylaxis may be started in patients where it is anticipated.

Ovarian hyperstimulation syndrome should be avoided as it can lead to further compromise in renal function due to the intravascular hypovolemia and mechanical pressure of the enlarged ovaries on the transplanted organs.

In 2015, Normann et al. observed postrenal transplant patients undergoing IVF for long-term outcomes. They compared the singletons and twins with corresponding singletons and twins in singleton pregnancies in post-transplant patients.[20]

Among the fetal outcomes observed, there was a significant higher morbidity in the neonatal and early neonatal periods. A significantly higher infant mortality was also observed in post-transplant IVF patients. Although the incidence of birth defects showed a similar incidence, the observed mean age at follow-up of the children was 14.7 years.[21]

There was a higher incidence of acute bronchitis, systemic lupus erythematosus, and hyperactivity disorders in children delivered to women with renal transplantation than in children delivered to women with no transplanted organs. Otherwise, long-term child morbidity was comparable.

TRANSPLANT INTERNATIONAL REGISTRY

Transplant International Registry was a program founded by Dr Vincent Armenti in 1991. Although initially a national program, it later became an international registry, including data from 25 other countries. They have collected data on 1,836 post-transplant patients. They follow-up the post-transplant pregnant patients, and even 250 grandchildren have also been included in the list.

The registry works towards formulation of standards of care of pregnancy and contraception amongst transplant recipients. One of the most important components of successful outcomes following pregnancy is a multidisciplinary regulated approach for the management of such patients.[18,21]

KEY LEARNING POINTS

- Patients with a renal transplant as recipients should be treated as high-risk pregnancies.
- A multidisciplinary team approach is to be followed for management of such patients. The initial counseling should begin in the peritransplant phase.
- A thorough preconception evaluation, which also includes management of immunosuppression and explaining the risks and likely complications, should be done with the patient and family.
- Overall, these patients have a good fertility, and the outcomes following pregnancy are favorable if the graft function preconception is stable.

■ REFERENCES

1. Humphreys RA, Wong HH, Milner R, Matsuda-Abedini M. Pregnancy outcomes among solid organ transplant recipients in British Columbia. J Obstet Gynaecol Can. 2012;34(5):416-24.
2. Saha MT, Saha HH, Niskanen LK, Salmela KT, Pasternack AI. Time course of serum prolactin and sex hormones following successful renal transplantation. Nephron. 2002;92(3):735-7.
3. Yaprak M, Doğru V, Sanhal CY, Özgür K, Erman M. In vitro fertilization after renal transplantation: a single-center experience. Transplant Proc. 2019;51(4):1089-92.
4. Bailie GR, Elder SJ, Mason NA, Asano Y, Cruz JM, Fukuhara S, et al. Sexual dysfunction in dialysis patients treated with antihypertensive or antidepressive medications: results from the DOPPS. Nephrol Dial Transplant. 2007;22(4):1163-70.
5. Anantharaman P, Schmidt RJ. Sexual function in chronic kidney disease. Adv Chronic Kidney Dis. 2007;14:119-25.
6. Perri A, Izzo G, Lofaro D, La Vignera S, Brunetti A, Calogero AE, et al. Erectile dysfunction after kidney transplantation. J Clin Med. 2020;9(6):1991.
7. Wang GC, Zheng JH, Xu LG, Min ZL, Zhu YH, Qi J, et al. Measurements of serum pituitary-gonadal hormones and investigation of sexual and reproductive functions in kidney transplant recipients. Int J Nephrol. 2010;2010:612126.
8. Murray JE, Reid DE, Harrison JH, Merrill JP. Successful pregnancies after human renal transplantation. N Engl J Med. 1963;269:341-3.
9. Shah S, Venkatesan RL, Gupta A, Sanghavi MK, Welge J, Johansen R, et al. Pregnancy outcomes in women with kidney transplant: metaanalysis and systematic review. BMC Nephrol. 2019;20(1):24.

10. Deshpande NA, James NT, Kucirka LM, Boyarsky BJ, Garonzik-Wang JM, Montgomery RA, et al. Pregnancy outcomes in kidney transplant recipients: a systematic review and meta-analysis. Am J Transplant. 2011;11(11):2388-404.
11. Kainz A, Harabacz I, Cowlrick IS, Gadgil SD, Hagiwara D. Review of the course and outcome of 100 pregnancies in 84 women treated with tacrolimus. Transplantation. 2000;70(12):1718-21.
12. Deshpande NA, James NT, Kucirka LM, Boyarsky BJ, Garonzik-Wang JM, Cameron AM, et al. Pregnancy outcome of liver transplant recipients: a systematic review and meta-analysis. Liver Transpl. 2012;18:621-9.
13. Sarkar M, Bramham K, Moritz MJ, Coscia L. Reproductive health in women following abdominal organ transplant. Am J Transplant. 2018;18(5):1068-76.
14. Cabiddu G, Spotti D, Gernone G, Santoro D, Moroni G, Gregorini G, et al. A best-practice position statement on pregnancy after kidney transplantation: focusing on the unsolved questions. The Kidney and Pregnancy Study Group of the Italian Society of Nephrology. J Nephrol. 2018;31(5):665-81.
15. Klein CL, Josephson MA. Post-transplant pregnancy and contraception. Clin J Am Soc Nephrol. 2022;17(1):114-20.
16. Hebert MF, Zheng S, Hays K, Shen DD, Davis CL, Umans JG, et al. Interpreting tacrolimus concentrations during pregnancy and postpartum. Transplantation. 2013;95(7):908-15.
17. Majak GB, Sandven I, Lorentzen B, Vangen S, Reisaeter AV, Henriksen T, et al. Pregnancy outcomes following maternal kidney transplantation: a national cohort study. Acta Obstet Gynecol Scand. 2016;95:1153-61.
18. Ohler L, Coscia L, Armenti V. Milestones in transplantation. Prog Transplant. 2008;18:63-4.
19. Lockwood GM, Ledger WL, Barlow DH. Successful pregnancy outcome in a renal transplant patient following in-vitro fertilization. Hum Reprod. 1995;10:1528-30.
20. Norrman E, Bergh C, Wennerholm UB. Pregnancy outcome and long-term follow-up after in vitro fertilization in women with renal transplantation. Hum Reprod. 2015;30(1):205-13.
21. Coscia L, Constantinescu S, Moritz MJ. 347.12: Transplant Pregnancy Registry International - 30 Years of Data Collection. Transplantation. 2022;106(9S):S360.

Assisted Reproductive Technology in Postliver Transplant

Vidhi Chaudhary, Pikee Saxena

■ INTRODUCTION

Solid organ transplantation is the final approach to increase longevity in women with end-stage diseases involving the kidney, liver, lung, heart, and pancreas. An imbalance in the hypothalamic–pituitary–ovarian axis in women with chronic renal failure or severe hepatic dysfunction results in anovulation and reduced fertility.[1,2] Due to innovations in solid organ transplantation, there has been improvement in survival of transplant recipients. This has led to an increased in quality of life, desire to conceive, and subsequently having a healthy live birth. Most often, fertility is restored with successful organ transplantation with overall good health.[3]

The first successful deceased donor liver transplant in India was done in 1998, shortly followed by the first successful living donor liver transplant in November 1998.[4,5]

Postliver transplant there is improvement in subfertility in majority (70-95%) of the patients.[5,6] In women with persistent subfertility, important causes are usually liver related, i.e., usage of immunosuppressants, varying degrees of liver dysfunction, postliver transplant development of abdominal adhesions leading to the tubal blockage, portosystemic shunting of androgens, and disordered metabolism of sex hormones. Other nonliver-related factors may include primary reproductive disorders, advanced maternal age, and depression. Chronic liver disease and malnutrition can also affect fertility in these women.[6,7] Due to these factors, women of childbearing age usually consider assisted conception after conventional treatment methods have failed. The process of in vitro fertilization (IVF) and its potential impact on liver disease is yet to be understood. This chapter deals with the approach to infertility in the postliver transplant female recipients with the application of assisted reproductive technologies (ARTs) in achieving pregnancy with healthy live birth.[8] The foremost aim is to plan the pregnancy with the lowest risk of rejection, while on maintenance doses of immunosuppressants. In the USA, approximately 14,000 women of reproductive age undergo liver transplant whereas in the UK, there are approximately 12 pregnancies in liver transplant recipients per year.[9]

■ PRECONCEPTIONAL COUNSELING

Worldwide, 20–30% of patients are in reproductive age post solid-organ transplantation. The estimated rate of infertility is marginally higher in this group when compared with the general population.[10] A minimum gap of 2 years is required prior to conception in order to optimize maternal and fetal outcomes. Studies have shown that a transplant-to-conception interval of >2 years is associated with decreased rates of low birth weight (LBW), graft rejection, and graft loss.[11]

Prior to embarking on pregnancy, there must be a detailed discussion on the process of infertility treatment and its related complications including pregnancy-related care.

The effect of immunosuppression on the health of both mother and baby must be discussed in detail. It must be emphasized that immunosuppressive therapy is required to maintain adequate graft function during pregnancy and hence outweigh the possible associated fetal exposure risks. Therapeutic and lowest possible required doses of immunosuppression prior to and during pregnancy are key in preventing complications in both mother and fetus. Maintenance of preconception immunosuppression is generally recommended, except for mycophenolate mofetil (MMF).[12]

Common medical comorbidities such as diabetes and hypertension must be optimized prior to embarking on any fertility-related treatment. Mental health research shows that female graft recipients reportedly have a higher risk of postnatal depression and a reduced quality of life. Therefore, psychological assessment should form an integral part of infertility treatment.[10]

Vaccinations: Influenza, pneumococcal, hepatitis B, and tetanus vaccination must be completed prepregnancy. Rubella and varicella vaccination must be preferably completed 12 weeks prior to pregnancy.[6]

Preconceptionally, folic acid is to be advised.

Immunosuppressants

Immunosuppressive therapy during pregnancy maintains adequate graft function, thereby resulting in successful obstetric outcomes. Immunosuppressants which are contraindicated in pregnancy need to be switched to a safer alternative.[13,14] The overview of immunosuppressants in pregnancy is given in the following text.

Mycophenolate Mofetil

Mycophenolate mofetil is an absolute contraindication in pregnancy. Potential risks include spontaneous abortion (49%), structural anomalies (23%), and stillbirth (2%). Reported literature shows a high incidence of malformations, including cleft lip/palate abnormalities, hypoplastic nails, shortened fifth fingers, and microtia. Patients are advised to ideally use two methods of contraception for a minimum of 4 weeks prior to initiating MMF, during MMF treatment, and for 12 weeks after discontinuation of MMF.[6,12-14]

Corticosteroids

Around 10% of the maternal corticosteroid dose is transferred via placenta to fetus. Newer studies do not demonstrate any evidence of teratogenicity of corticosteroids; hence, they are safe during pregnancy. Repeated or prolonged exposure of systemic corticosteroids in pregnancy has reportedly been associated with fetal growth restriction (FGR). Short courses of corticosteroids used for fetal lung maturation in threatened preterm deliveries are likely to be safe and are recommended.[15]

Azathioprine

Azathioprine as an immunosuppressant is considered safe during pregnancy. It readily crosses the placenta, but the fetal liver lacks inosinate pyrophosphorylase, which is the key enzyme required to convert azathioprine into its active form. Lymphopenia, thymic hypoplasia, and hypogammaglobulinemia have been seen in children born to mothers on immunosuppression with azathioprine.

These changes, however, are temporary and usually reverse after birth with no future long-term consequences being so far reported.

There are studies showing dose-related myelosuppression in the fetus, but maintenance of mother's white cell count >7,500 mm^3 appears to reduce this risk.[16,17]

Cyclosporine

Current literature indicates that there is no increased risk of congenital malformations when compared with nonexposed women. Cyclosporine readily crosses the placenta with fetal blood concentrations reaching between 30% and 60% of the mother's concentration. However, this predisposes the fetus to a moderate risk of FGR. Hence, pregnant postliver transplant women on cyclosporine immunosuppression must be monitored via serial growth scans. Hepatic cytochrome P450 enzymes can be altered during pregnancy, leading to changes in drug distribution, hepatic clearance, and renal dysfunction. Cyclosporine levels must be serially measured during pregnancy in order to prevent toxicity or underdosing.[16,18]

Tacrolimus

Tacrolimus is considered safe in pregnancy but requires close monitoring of its serum levels by the transplant team. Nephrotoxicity and glucose intolerance during pregnancy in association with tacrolimus use have been reported. Interestingly, reduced incidences of preeclampsia and hypertension have been seen compared to cyclosporine-based therapy. Reversible, transient, unexplained hyperkalemia not requiring treatment has been noted in newborns of mothers taking tacrolimus.[18] The rate of malformations is around 4–5% in liver transplant recipients and hence comparable to the general population.[18,19]

ASSISTED REPRODUCTIVE TECHNOLOGY IN POSTLIVER TRANSPLANT WOMEN

In postliver transplant female recipients, there are imperative medical, psychosocial, and ethical concerns involved in treating fertility-related issues. Hence, it is logical to involve a multidisciplinary team involving ART specialist, reproductive endocrinologists, transplant physician, hepatologists, and obstetricians to ensure a successful ART and pregnancy outcome without compromising graft function or maternal health. The primary aim of ART is to achieve singleton pregnancy while avoiding complications, such as ovarian hyperstimulation syndrome (OHSS), that pose greater risks in transplant recipients. Liver transplantation may prolong the life expectancy of patients with the end-stage liver disease; there is little clinical experience with such patients requiring controlled ovarian stimulation and IVF. Infertility diagnosis and workup in liver transplant patients are similar to the general population. Application of ARTs is reasonable and gives favorable outcomes if patients are managed rationally, with careful attention to prevention of iatrogenic complications.[20]

In Vitro Fertilization Cycle Consideration

IVF treatment's success depends on factors such as current graft function, woman's age, and, most importantly, her ovarian reserve. Reproductive potential diminishes with age due to reduced quality of oocytes and their genetic material. There is a trend of higher proportion of live birth rate (LBR) in women who conceived more than 1 year after liver transplantation than in women who conceived prior to 1 year. Tacrolimus exposure is associated with higher risks of premature delivery and cesarean section than cyclosporine exposure.[14] The overall average implantation rate per IVF cycle is 60.8% for liver transplant recipients.[6] 70% of the women who conceive after liver transplantation have successful live births; however, this rate is lower than that of women in the general population.

Usually, a long protocol has been used involving gonadotrophin-releasing hormone (GnRH) agonist suppression of the cycle followed by step-up gonadotrophin regimen in case reports published in literature on ART in postliver transplant women. Starting dose, however, has been extrapolated from clinical case reports which is usually 150 IU follicle-stimulating hormone (FSH) or better to be individualized. Monitoring is done by ultrasonography (USG) till desired dominant follicles of 18 mm are achieved. Transvaginal oocyte retrieval is done 36–48 hours after inj. human chorionic gonadotropin trigger of 5,000–10,000 IU. Single-embryo transfer (SET) at the blastocyst stage is preferred in postliver transplant patients to mitigate the risk of high-order pregnancy in double-embryo transfer as these women already have an increased risk of hypertension in pregnancy, preeclampsia, preterm delivery, and small for gestational age (SGA) babies.[8,20,21]

The aim of controlled ovarian stimulation (COS) is to minimize the risk of complications, i.e., OHSS, multiple pregnancy, and thromboembolism. So, all precautions are taken during stimulation to avoid the risk of OHSS, and SET is preferred to avoid the risk of multiple pregnancies and their related complications. These women should be advised to remain well hydrated. Mechanical deep-vein thrombosis (DVT) prophylaxis to be used and risk assessment to be done if they need low-molecular weight heparin (LMWH).

Gonadotrophin-releasing hormone (GnRH) antagonists, either as fixed or as flexible protocol, are another option in these patients as a recent Cochrane review has opined its efficacy in preventing a luteinizing hormone (LH) surge during a controlled ovarian hyperstimulation (COH) without the hypoestrogenic side effects, flare-up, or long downregulation period associated with agonists. Also, they have a lower incidence of OHSS which has a benefit in postliver transplant women.[22]

Complications of In Vitro Fertilization

Ovarian hyperstimulation syndrome is a rare complication of an IVF cycle. It is an exaggerated response to a superovulation cycle giving rise to a varied spectrum of excessive ovarian enlargement, hypovolemia, hemoconcentration, acute shifting of fluid into extravascular spaces (ascites and pleural effusions), and electrolyte imbalance. There is limited data on the effects of IVF therapy in postliver transplant women. Due to supraphysiological concentration of estrogen, there is hypercoagulability and hemoconcentration causing microvascular thrombosis and tissue ischemia leading to microvascular leak and fluid shift. Direct estrogen/progesterone effects lead to induction of enzymes causing hepatocellular damage.

One small study reported a prevalence of (7.1%) OHSS. As per the study, there was no hepatic decompensation and postpartum flare of the damage was usually mild which improved after the resolution of OHSS.[23] However, abnormal liver enzymes during an IVF cycle may be associated with decreased rates of pregnancy.[17] Excessive ovarian stimulation may increase the risk of liver failure later in pregnancy, as an after effect of IVF. IVF increases the risk of hypertensive disorders of pregnancy and its complications such as hemolysis, elevated liver enzymes, and low platelet syndrome (HELLP).[24]

OBSTETRIC CONCERNS IN POSTLIVER TRANSPLANT WOMEN

Pregnant liver transplant recipients need a multidisciplinary team approach which includes an obstetrician, a liver transplant surgeon, and a hepatologist. Post successful liver transplantation, an interval of at least 12-24 months is recommended before embarking on the pregnancy. Immunosuppressants must be reviewed prepregnancy. Overall, the risk of adverse outcomes in pregnancy is higher for liver transplant patients when compared with the background population but lower than that for renal transplant recipients. In addition to general obstetric care, the following must be done:[8,24]

- *First trimester:* Full blood count, urea and electrolytes, serum iron, vitamin D levels, viral infection screen [toxoplasma, cytomegalovirus (CMV), hepatitis B/C, and human immunodeficiency virus (HIV)], and viability scan to be carried out. Review vaccinations as stated above.
- Consider low-dose aspirin prophylaxis from 12 weeks onward.
- Vitamin D deficiency, as per medical literature, is associated with an increased rate of preeclampsia and hence, supplementation is recommended from the first trimester.
- Early screening of diabetes in the first trimester (if screen negative, repeat at 24-28 weeks of gestation) and hypertension is required once pregnancy is achieved.
- Screening of FGR with serial growth scans at 28, 32, and 36 weeks of gestation is required.
- Planned delivery either via cesarean section or induction of labor is key to reducing the risk of obstetric-related complications.
- Monthly—consider CMV levels
- Monthly—obstetric review and hepatology review for graft function
- Monitor serum cyclosporine and tacrolimus levels in each trimester to check graft function.

Maternal Outcomes[9,25-27]

- *Graft rejection:* The prevalence of acute rejection is 0-20% and graft loss within the first 2 years of pregnancy is around 10.5%. This data is not matched for nonpregnant liver transplant recipients. It remains unclear whether these events are a direct cause of pregnancy itself. Rates of postpartum graft rejection range between 3 and 12%.
- *Infections:* The frequency of infections acquired during pregnancy in liver transplant recipients has similar preponderance to that of the general population by around 11%.
- *Anemia:* It is a common complication in pregnant liver transplant recipients. It is secondary to physiological changes during pregnancy,

effects of immunosuppression, renal insufficiency, and iron deficiency. The reported prevalence is 23%.
- *Gestational diabetes mellitus (GDM):* Pregnancy is a physiological state of insulin resistance. Diabetogenic immunosuppressants, along with the presence of additional risk factors, may cause the development of GDM. The reported rates of GDM in pregnant liver transplant recipients vary between 0 and 11%. Hence, early screening for gestational diabetes mellitus (GDM) is advocated. There are reports of increased rates of cholestasis of pregnancy and increased preeclampsia (10-16.8%) in liver transplant recipients.

Fetal Outcomes[9,27,28]

- *LBR:* In postliver transplant women recipients, LBR is reported between 65% and 77%. The miscarriage rate has been reported to be between 5.4% and 11.1% which is similar to general population.
- *Congenital infections:* Recurrent CMV infection in the immunosuppressed female patient is known to cause congenital CMV infection. If untreated, this can cause serious fetal complications such as hydrops fetalis, stillbirth, mental retardation, visual/hearing loss, prematurity, or death. It is therefore important to monitor CMV levels during pregnancy in liver transplant recipients when indicated.[29]
- *FGR:* FGR rates in liver transplant recipients are increased when compared with the general population and so is the rate of preterm delivery (39-42%), LBW babies (16-21%), and cesarean delivery (35.2-49.6%). Serial growth scans should be done at 26-28 weeks, 32-34 weeks, and 36 weeks of gestation, respectively, for early detection of FGR and instituting appropriate management. Kamarajah et al. reported higher risks of premature birth delivery and increased rates of cesarean section in women on tacrolimus therapy during pregnancy as compared to cyclosporine.[15,26] In addition, women with liver transplants, with coexisting chronic kidney disease, have poorer pregnancy outcomes.[30]

■ POSTPARTUM PHASE AND BREASTFEEDING

After childbirth, there is return of all parameters to normal physiological levels, which may lead to an alteration of immunosuppressant levels and hence its recommended to monitor their levels if readjustments are required.

Postpartum special consideration should be made to prevent thromboembolism including adequate hydration, early mobilization, and thromboprophylaxis, wherever needed.

Breastfeeding is not an absolute contraindication. Informed choice must be offered to adequately assess and weigh the potential risks of drug exposure versus the benefits of breastfeeding, i.e., reduced rates of allergies, infections, and colitis. It is safe to breastfeed in case of low doses of corticosteroids, azathioprine, and tacrolimus. However, breastfeeding with cyclosporine must be done with caution due to concerns about possible immunosuppression in the infant. Hence, drug levels must be monitored. Breastfed infants should be monitored if this drug is used during lactation, possibly including measurement of serum levels to rule out toxicity if there is a concern.[31-33]

■ CONCLUSION

Solid organ transplantation is key for improving quality of life for end-stage liver disease. With innovations in medical research, women with postliver transplantation are able to achieve healthy reproductive outcomes. Multidisciplinary approach, stable liver function, use of appropriate pregnancy friendly immunosuppressants, intake of multivitamins, proper diet and regular antenatal and postnatal surveillance leads to healthy maternal and neonatal outcomes.

KEY LEARNING POINTS

- A multidisciplinary team is required in the counseling and monitoring of liver transplant recipients both before and during pregnancy.
- ART is relatively safe in postliver transplant women with stable liver function.
- All liver transplantation recipients should wait for a minimum of 2 years before embarking on pregnancy for healthy outcomes.
- MMF must be stopped in those planning to conceive and should be switched to safer immunosuppressants.
- Preconceptionally, folic acid is advised and vaccinations against influenza, pneumococcal, hepatitis B, tetanus, varicella, and rubella must be completed.
- Low-dose aspirin and vitamin D supplementation should begin from 12 weeks onwards.
- Serum cyclosporine and tacrolimus levels must be monitored in each trimester to assess graft function.
- Serial ultrasound monitoring to assess for FGR is required.
- Special attention should be given to obstetric complications such as hypertension, preeclampsia, FGR, and preterm delivery.
- Liver transplant recipients have relatively healthy neonatal with delivery of term and normal birth weight babies.
- In the postpartum period, thromboprophylaxis assessment should be considered.
- It is safe to breastfeed in case of low doses of corticosteroids, azathioprine, and tacrolimus. However, monitoring of breastfed neonates by measuring drug levels for toxicity must be considered.
- There is a paucity of high-quality randomized controlled trials on pregnancy in transplantation. This mandates the collection of accurate and reliable data through active national and international registries.

■ REFERENCES

1. Zullo F, Saccone G, Donnarumma L, Marino I, Guida M, Berghella V. Pregnancy after liver transplantation: a case series and review of the literature. J Matern Fetal Neonatal Med. 2021;34(19):3269-76.

2. Douglas NC, Shah M, Sauer M. Fertility and reproductive disorders in female solid organ transplant recipients. Semin Perinatol. 2007;31(6):332-8.
3. Mass K, Quint EH, Punch MR, Merion RM. Gynecological and reproductive function after liver transplantation. Transplantation 1996;62(4):476-9.
4. Poonacha P, Sibal A, Soin AS, Rajashekar MR, Rajakumari DV. India's first successful pediatric liver transplant. Indian Pediatr. 2001;38(3):287-91.
5. Narasimhan G. Living donor liver transplantation in India. Hepatobiliary Surg Nutr. 2016;5(2):127-32.
6. Rahim MN, Long L, Penna L, Williamson C, Kametas NA, Nicolaides KH, et al. Pregnancy in liver transplantation. Liver Transpl. 2020;26(4):564-85.
7. Burra P, Germani G, Masier A, De Martin E, Gambato M, Salonia A, et al. Sexual dysfunction in chronic liver disease: is liver transplantation an effective cure? Transplantation. 2010;89:1425-9.
8. Case AM, Weissman A, Sermer M, Greenblatt EM. Successful twin pregnancy in a dual-transplant couple resulting from in vitro fertilization and intracytoplasmic sperm injection: case report. Hum Reprod. 2000;15(3):626-8.
9. Marzec I, Słowakiewicz A, Gozdowska J, Tronina O, Pacholczyk M, Lisik W, et al. Pregnancy after liver transplant: maternal and perinatal outcomes. BMC Pregnancy Childbirth. 2021;21:627.
10. Ulug U, Mesut A, Jozwiak EA, Bahceci M. Successful pregnancy in a liver transplant recipient following controlled ovarian hyperstimulation and intracytoplasmic sperm injection. J Assist Reprod Genet. 2005;22(7):311-3.
11. Szymusik I, Warzecha D, Wielgoś M, Pietrzak B. Infertility in female and male solid organ recipients - from diagnosis to treatment: an up-to-date review of the literature. Ann Transplant. 2020;25:e9235921-8.
12. Blume C, Pischke S, Von Versen-Höynck F, Günter HH, Gross MM. Pregnancies in liver and kidney transplant recipients: a review of the current literature and recommendation. Best Pract Res Clin Obstet Gynaecol. 2014;28(8):1123-36.
13. Sifontis NM, Coscia LA, Constantinescu S, Lavelanet AF, Moritz MJ, Armenti VT. Pregnancy outcomes in solid organ transplant recipients with exposure to mycophenolate mofetil or sirolimus. Transplantation. 2006;82:1698-702.
14. Kim M, Rostas S, Gabardi S. Mycophenolate fetal toxicity and risk evaluation and mitigation strategies. Am J Transplant 2013;13(6):1383-9.
15. Kamarajah SK, Arntdz K, Bundred J, Gunson B, Haydon G, Thompson F. Outcomes of pregnancy in recipients of liver transplants. Clin Gastroenterol Hepatol. 2019;17(7):1398-404.
16. Skuladottir H, Wilcox AJ, Ma C, Lammer EJ, Rasmussen SA, Werler MM, et al. Corticosteroid use and risk of orofacial clefts. Birth Defects Res A Clin Mol Teratol. 2014;100:499-506.
17. Casanova MJ, Chaparro M, Domenech E, Barreiro-De Acosta M, Bermejo F, Iglesias E, et al. Safety of thiopurines and anti-TNF-α drugs during pregnancy in patients with inflammatory bowel disease. Am J Gastroenterol 2013;108:433-40.
18. Angelberger S, Reinisch W, Messerschmidt A, Miehsler W, Novacek G, Vogelsang H, et al. Long-term follow-up of babies exposed to azathioprine in utero and via breastfeeding. J Crohns Colitis. 2011;5:95-100.
19. Kainz A, Harabacz I, Cowlrick IS, Gadgil S, Hagiwara D. Analysis of 100 pregnancy outcomes in women treated systemically with tacrolimus. Transpl Int. 2000;13:S299-300.

20. Coscia LA, Constantinescu S, Moritz MJ, Frank AM, Ramirez CB, Maley WR, et al. Report from the National Transplantation Pregnancy Registry (NTPR): outcomes of pregnancy after transplantation. Clin Transplant. 2010;65-85.
21. Rahim MN, Theocharidou E, Yen Lau KG, Ahmed R, Marattukalam F, Long L, et al. Safety and efficacy of in vitro fertilisation in patients with chronic liver disease and liver transplantation recipients. J Hepatol. 2021;74(6):1407-15.
22. Choi JM, Mahany EB, Sauer MV. Pregnancy after in vitro fertilization in a liver transplant patient. Reprod Med Biol. 2012;12(2):69-70.
23. Al-Inany HG, Youssef MA, Ayeleke RO, Brown J, Lam WS, Broekmans FJ. Gonadotrophin-releasing hormone antagonists for assisted reproductive technology. Cochrane Database Syst Rev. 2016;4(4):CD001750.
24. Forman RG, Frydman R, Egan D, Ross C, Barlow DH. Severe ovarian hyperstimulation syndrome using agonists of gonadotropin-releasing hormone for in vitro fertilization: a European series and a proposal for prevention. Fertil Steril. 1990;53:502-9.
25. Giugliano E, Cagnazzo E, Pansini G, Vesce F, Marci R. Ovarian stimulation and liver dysfunction: is a clinical relationship possible? A case of hepatic failure after repeated cycles of ovarian stimulation. Clin Exp Reprod Med. 2013;40:38-41.
26. Marson EJ, Kamarajah SK, Dyson JK, White SA. Pregnancy outcomes in women with liver transplants: systematic review and meta-analysis. HPB (Oxford). 2020;22(8):1102-11.
27. Christopher V, Al-Chalabi T, Richardson PD, Mulesan P, Rela M, Heaton ND, et al. Pregnancy outcome after liver transplantation: a single-center experience of 71 pregnancies in 45 recipients. Liver Transpl. 2006;12(7):1138-43.
28. Wijarnpreecha K, Thongprayoon C, Sanguankeo A, Upala S, Ungprasert P, Cheungpasitporn W. Hepatitis C infection and intrahepatic cholestasis of pregnancy: a systematic review and meta-analysis. Clin Res Hepatol Gastroenterol. 2017;41:39-45.
29. Prodromidou A, Kostakis ID, Machairas N, Garoufalia Z, Stamopoulos P, Paspala A, et al. Pregnancy outcomes after liver transplantation: a systematic review. Transplant Proc. 2019;51(2):446-9.
30. Ross DS, Dollard SC, Victor M, Sumartojo E, Cannon MJ. The epidemiology and prevention of congenital cytomegalovirus infection and disease: activities of the centers for disease control and prevention workgroup. J Womens Health (Larchmt). 2006;15(3):224-9.
31. Mohamed-Ahmed O, Nelson-Piercy C, Bramham K, Gao H, Kurinczuk JJ, Brocklehurst P, et al. Pregnancy outcomes in liver and cardiothoracic transplant recipients: A UK National Cohort Study. PLoS One. 2014;9(2):e89151.
32. Flint J, Panchal S, Hurrell A, van de Venne M, Gayed M, Schreiber K, et al. BSR and BHPR guideline on prescribing drugs in pregnancy and breastfeeding-Part I: standard and biologic disease modifying anti-rheumatic drugs and corticosteroids. Rheumatol (United Kingdom). 2016;55:1693-7.
33. Constantinescu S, Pai A, Coscia LA, Davison JM, Moritz MJ, Armenti VT. Breast-feeding after transplantation. Best Pract Res Clin Obstet Gynaecol. 2014;28:1163-73.

Male Fertility and Solid Organ Transplants

Vineet Malhotra, Vilvapathy Senguttuvan Karthikeyan, Priyank Kothari

■ INTRODUCTION

Male infertility is on the rise.[1] There are multiple causes of male infertility, including varicocele, hormonal problems such as hypogonadism, genetic causes, and drugs. Further, chronic medical conditions or their treatment can affect sperms and cause infertility. Out of these, chronic kidney disease (CKD) and chronic liver disease (CLD) play an important role in male infertility. The treatment in the form of transplant improves the situation but still can be associated with effects leading to infertility. This chapter addresses the fertility issues associated with chronic kidney and liver disease and transplantation.

■ CHRONIC KIDNEY DISEASE

Chronic kidney disease is becoming more prevalent. It is found that up to 40% of transplant recipients are constituted by men and women in their fertile period.[2] At this point, enough impetus to fertility and reproductive care is not provided at all centers. Coupled with an increasing prevalence of CKD in women and men of reproductive age, the importance of understanding fertility and reproductive technologies in this population cannot be understated. CKD can lead to problems in reproductive hormonal milieu due to uremia and inflammation. It is seen that CKD can be the cause of infertility in up to 15% of couples even before end-stage renal disease (ESRD) sets in.[3] With the long waiting list or paucity of organ availability, ESRD and its problems in these young patients are only worsening. The cause of infertility in men undergoing dialysis and due to associated or causative diabetes mellitus and hypertension is being explored. This is multifactorial; it can be due to CKD per se or other factors which need to be identified. CKD can lead to problems in sperm parameters, male reproductive hormones, and erectile function.[1]

Effect of Chronic Kidney Disease on Male Hormones

The main cause of hormonal imbalance is a change in the hypothalamic–pituitary–gonadal (HPG) axis owing to CKD. The exact etiopathogenesis is unknown; however, this seems to be due to disruption in the pulsatile release of gonadotropin-releasing hormone (GnRH) from the hypothalamus.[4]

It is also observed that testosterone levels are inversely related to interleukin-6, which is a proinflammatory cytokine elevated in CKD.[5] With reduced GnRH release, luteinizing hormone (LH) levels are altered and so are the testosterone levels. This is coupled with Leydig cell dysfunction associated with CKD and more with ESRD, which worsens the hypogonadism.[6] The other important factor disturbing reproductive hormones, especially testosterone levels, is the high level of prolactin (PRL) in CKD men. This elevated PRL offsets the proper functioning of the HPG axis. Hyperprolactinemia is proposed to be due to reduced renal clearance and loss of negative feedback.[7] There is also evidence of Sertoli cell dysfunction, marked by lowered anti-Müllerian hormone (AMH) levels in men. This, in addition to the quoted Leydig cell dysfunction, overall leads to sperm dysfunction. There is also a state of hypergonadotropic hypogonadism in men with CKD.[8,9] It has been shown that renal transplantation has been effective in reversing this pathology. In addition, because of Leydig cell dysfunction, free testosterone levels are often low. The low testosterone level results in an increase in LH and a reduced and delayed response to human chorionic gonadotropin (hCG) stimulation.[9] Serum LH and testosterone levels get normalized after transplant, and sperm parameters do improve.[6,7] A circulating LH receptor inhibitor has been implicated in Leydig cell resistance and impaired feedback mechanism.[10] Uremia leads to reduced urinary LH excretion resulting in high serum LH levels, combined with less bioactive forms.[11] Hyperprolactinemia in renal insufficiency is partially induced by a decreased metabolic clearance but also by autonomic overproduction.[12]

End-stage Renal Disease and Sperm Parameters

Renal failure by itself can worsen sperm parameters due to uremia.[1] There may be associated erectile dysfunction (ED), and this can also be due to hormonal imbalance associated with CKD. Men with CKD have reduced ejaculate volume, oligozoospermia, reduced sperm motility, and reduced sperms with normal morphology.[13] They have poorly viable sperms. On long term, fibrosis sets in these testes, and histopathology may show impaired germ cell proliferation and Sertoli cell atrophy.[14] Testis volume continues to worsen in men undergoing hemodialysis.[15] Out of all these parameters, motility and sperm morphology are the most affected in CKD. Sperms in CKD men have acrosome, head, and tail defects.[16] It has also been observed that cystic fibrosis transmembrane conductance regulatory gene levels are reduced in men with CKD, irrespective of infertility.[17]

Further, in younger men, CKD may be associated with congenital kidney anomalies. As the development of the genitourinary system happens simultaneously, these men may be predisposed to infertility. Posterior urethral valves are associated with erectile or ejaculatory dysfunction.

Congenital unilateral or bilateral absence of vas deferens can be picked up in these young men, where the cause is likely to be obstructive.[18-20]

In adolescent males, it has been shown time and again that transplantation in young ages has good outcomes on testis volume, sperm parameters, and fertility.[1,21] Uremia at the time of puberty can lead to irreversible damage to testis, a state of hypergonadotropic hypogonadism, and there has been multifold improvement in sperm parameters postrenal transplant.[1]

Erectile Dysfunction in Chronic Kidney Disease

Erectile dysfunction in CKD is multifactorial.[1] It can be due to diabetes mellitus or hypertension; effect of uremia, drugs such as beta blockers, neuromodulators, and diuretics used in CKD patients; and the extreme stress and anxiety associated with the medical condition and treatment.[1,22] It is of importance to identify the cause of ED and its effect. ED may be a singular cause of infertility in couples with normal hormones and semen parameters. Postrenal transplant, the improvement is widely variable, ranging from nil up to 75%.[23]

Effect of Immunosuppression Used During Renal Transplantation

Along with CKD and renal transplant, immunosuppressive drugs used for renal transplantation also have an effect on male fertility.[1] Out of calcineurin inhibitors, tacrolimus has minimal sperm damage.[24] Sirolimus and cyclosporine can cause oligoasthenoteratozoospermia and hypogonadism, and it affects testicular architecture. There are not many differences in hormonal levels between sirolimus and tacrolimus. mTOR (mechanistic target of rapamycin) inhibitors can lead to hypogonadism, oligoasthenoteratozoospermia, and reduced spontaneous pregnancy rates.[25,26] Mycophenolate mofetil inhibits deoxyribonucleic acid (DNA) synthesis and is reported to have teratogenic effects, but its effect on spermatogenesis is unknown.[27]

Effect of Renal Transplantation

During renal transplant recipient surgery, there is potential damage to vas deferens and vascular supply to the testis during transplant bed preparation in the retroperitoneum.[28] It is important to take utmost care to avoid damaging spermatic cord structures during the surgery.[29] Spermatogenesis definitely is shown to improve after renal transplant. However, this improvement was not universal. A significant proportion of men with azoospermia did not improve.[6] Comparing the sperm parameters in fertile and infertile men, before and after renal transplant, showed that oligoasthenospermia and flagellar defects were seen in the infertile men despite transplantation.[22]

Renal transplant itself can be considered as a therapeutic option for CKD-induced ED and male infertility. The beneficial effect from transplant on male infertility and semen parameters is highly variable. Maturation arrest and reduced spermatogenesis constitute the predominant histology before transplant. Number of spermatogonia, all forms of sperms, and mature sperms improve after renal transplantation, but late maturation arrest is less likely to improve due to permanent damage associated with CKD. Paternity rates appear to improve significantly following renal transplant.[30] Persistent oligoasthenozoospermia following renal transplant is an indication for assisted reproduction. These men benefit from additional workup and management including the use of intracytoplasmic sperm injection (ICSI).[31] Successful ICSI has been reported in unique male transplant recipients such as cystinosis and hyperoxaluria.[32,33]

Treatment of Hormonal Disturbances

Renal transplant has been found to improve testosterone levels by up to twice the preoperative levels. However, 40% of men had persistent hypogonadism after renal transplant. Follicle-stimulating hormone (FSH) and LH remain elevated in these men post kidney transplant, but estradiol and PRL do reduce significantly. Defects in gonadotropin at level of pituitary and hypothalamic function contribute to the impaired fertility observed in men and women with CKD, and this can be corrected by giving gonadotropins.[14] Men on dialysis have reduced numbers of mature spermatocytes, decreased sperm counts, and poorly functioning sperm, pointing to evidence of impaired spermatogenesis.[34] Sperm parameters do improve postrenal transplant. Nocturnal hemodialysis was shown to produce significant reduction in PRL and better testosterone levels, while LH and FSH were unchanged in a cohort of 30 men.[35] Men with CKD and hyperprolactinemia have reported benefit from bromocriptine and cabergoline, which are dopamine agonists aimed at reducing PRL levels.[12] Clomiphene citrate, a selective estrogen receptor modulator, has been shown to improve testosterone levels on hemodialysis and also LH and FSH levels.[36]

Treatment of Erectile Dysfunction in Chronic Kidney Disease

Phosphodiesterase-5 inhibitors (PDE5i) can be used for ED in renal modified dose. Tadalafil dosage has to be reduced based on the estimated glomerular filtration rate. In men with creatinine clearance (CrCl) <30 mL/min, tadalafil usage is not recommended while sildenafil can be used at 25 mg per oral dose.[37] They are effective in patients with mild-to-moderate ED.[38] In severe arteriogenic ED, self intracavernosal self-injections of vasoactive agents can be an option.[38] Testosterone can be used in men with sexual dysfunction (SD), not interested in fertility, and injections or transdermal preparations appear to have better testosterone levels. The role of platelet-rich plasma and low-intensity shockwave therapy is only experimental.[39]

■ LIVER DISEASE AND MALE FERTILITY

The causes for liver failure requiring liver transplantation are diverse, ranging from acute liver failure due to viral hepatitis, drug overdose, autoimmune hepatitis, and cirrhosis from chronic liver failure. The causes for CLD include chronic viral hepatitis, alcoholic liver disease, cholestatic liver disease, Budd–Chiari syndrome, and intrinsic hormonal deficiencies (storage disorders). Metabolic disorders include hyperoxaluria, amyloidosis, and urea cycle defects. Malignancies and polycystic liver disease patients can occasionally be candidates for liver transplant. The common spectrum among all diseases is decreased hepatic reserve and metabolic alterations. These affect the HPG axis at all levels and impair Leydig and Sertoli cell function.[40] There is a lot of stress and information coming up on the link of nonalcoholic fatty liver disease and metabolic syndrome with male SD and infertility.[41] The pathogenesis of reduced total and free testosterone combined with decreased LH levels is not fully understood.

Virus-induced chronic active hepatitis enhances oxidative stress in the reproductive system, aggravates sperm damage, and affects sperm quality parameters. The duration of hepatitis C virus (HCV) infection has correlated negatively with semen volume and sperm motility, while the viral load of HCV ribonucleic acid (RNA) has also negatively correlated with sperm concentration and motility. Also, men with chronic HCV infection have impaired hormonal function with lower testosterone and raised estradiol levels.[42] HCV also induces sperm DNA fragmentation.[43] Hepatitis B virus directly damages sperms and can integrate itself in the genome of sperm cells and vertically transmissible mutations, favoring apoptosis and necrosis.[44]

Influence of Liver Disease on Sexual Function

Liver failure is associated with an increased prevalence and severity of SD and is due to lower circulating testosterone levels, which may also be associated with alcohol intake.[45] The alterations in protein synthesis in the liver, favored by alcoholic cirrhosis and the often coexistent malnutrition, cooperate to alter the balance between linked (inactive) and available steroid hormones, with the final effect being a reduction in circulating androgens and an increase in estradiol levels in males, which has been considered detrimental for regular sexual function. Alcohol abuse is also associated with gastritis, pancreatitis, dilated cardiomyopathy, and brain atrophy, which all can be multifactorial causative factors for altered sexual condition.[46]

Improvement in Sexual Dysfunction and Semen Parameters Post-transplantation

Literature on pre- and postliver transplant semen parameters and sexual functioning is sparse. Reports state that there was an observed 4.8-fold rise for testosterone, 7.7-fold rise for free testosterone, and 3.4-fold rise for LH. Sexual function, endocrine status, and libido recovered as early as 6 weeks. The data on sperm parameters was too less to draw conclusions.[47] Future research is essential to prove the benefits of liver transplantation on sexual function and fertility.

Empirical Treatment of Erectile Dysfunction and Infertility in Liver Disease and Transplantation

Regarding PDE5i, no dose adjustment is required for sildenafil in mild-to-moderate liver failure (Child–Pugh classes A and B), while there is no evidence about its safe use in severe liver failure. Tadalafil can be used safely in mild-to-moderate liver failure and is effective.[48] Testosterone replacement therapy (TRT) in liver failure seems to be beneficial if there is no intent for future fertility. Though up to 90% of men with cirrhosis have testosterone deficiency, there is no clear evidence about TRT in these men. It has been found to improve muscle mass, bone mineral density, and anemia. TRT appears to be useful. Injectable preparations are better suited.[49] Testosterone levels seem to respond to clomifene citrate, which increases the FSH and LH levels indirectly, thus increasing testosterone levels. Oxidative stress is a common reason for several conditions associated with male infertility. High levels of reactive oxygen species (ROS) impair sperm quality by decreasing motility and increasing the oxidation of DNA, protein, and lipids. Multi-antioxidant supplementation is considered effective for male fertility parameters due to the synergistic effects of antioxidants. In liver failure, oxidative stress is induced due to generation of ROS and deficiency of liver enzymes responsible for counteracting these ROS, which occurs in the normal physiological state. This imbalance can be overcome by use of antioxidants, and this in turn leads to improvement in semen parameters and hence may lead to improvement in fertility. Folic acid, carnitine, arginine, and co-enzyme Q10 are the commonly used antioxidants which have shown benefit. Similar effects were reported with the use of *N*-acetylcysteine.[50] The treatment period is for around 3–6 months. Further evidence about liver transplant and treatment on male infertility and SD continues to evolve.

HEMATOPOIETIC AND OTHER SOLID ORGAN TRANSPLANTS AND MALE FERTILITY

Data on heart and lung transplant are scarce because of the more significant comorbidities, and patients are typically critically ill. Outcomes after transplant are promising, and reports are available that healthy children are born to these couples, with a 1.5-4% risk of congenital anomalies.[51] Similar outcomes are described in men undergoing hematopoietic cell transplant such as male infertility and SD due to sperm problems and testosterone deficiency. Routine screening for hypogonadism in asymptomatic men is not recommended. Spermatogenesis recovers 4 years after stopping cyclophosphamide therapy, and prevalence of nonobstructive azoospermia is reported to be as high as 85% after total body irradiation.[52] Fertility preservation is an important aspect in men undergoing treatment for these conditions, and sperm banking should ideally be discussed with all men who require fertility preservation.[53,54]

■ PRETRANSPLANT COUNSELING

It is vital to discuss about male infertility in men undergoing transplant. This includes evaluation of the male partner, duration of marital history and attempted conception, female partner factors such as age, comorbidities, and ovarian reserve, and about previous miscarriages, if any. Counseling should involve discussion about the chances of improvement with renal transplant, need for semen cryopreservation, possible effects of immunosuppressants, and the time available for the female partner for conception, in view of her ovarian reserve. Men may have SD, which could as well be addressed during this interview.

■ PRECONCEPTIONAL COUNSELING

In a male patient postrenal transplant on immunosuppression, it is important to have an informed discussion about the duration post-transplant after which the couple should start attempting for conception as immunosuppressants may affect fertility. The most commonly used maintenance immunosuppressants are calcineurin inhibitors, especially tacrolimus, mycophenolate mofetil, and corticosteroids for renal and liver transplant.[55,56] Calcineurin inhibitors possess certain properties that can adversely affect male fertility potential, but when used in the lowest possible doses to ensure proper renal allograft function, fertility is recovered after a period of 18-24 months from renal transplant. As this data is obtained from weak evidence, there are no recommendations regarding their use to optimize fertility.[25] Hence, a practical approach would be to have the patient on minimum dosages of immunosuppressants to maintain allograft function while semen analysis and hormone levels would guide the treatment. Initiating on medications such as antioxidants and planning for any interventions should be based on these reports. The couple should be assisted to take an informed decision regarding the same.

ASSISTED REPRODUCTION POST-TRANSPLANT

Semen parameters are reported to improve post-transplant and so is the fertility potential. The improvement may be marginal or significant. Immunosuppressants are known to affect sperm parameters, specifically counts and motility. The extent to which they affect the same varies as per the age of the patient, baseline semen parameters prior to transplant, and absence of any other secondary factors which may impair fertility potential. As time post-transplant increases, the level of immunosuppression decreases and hence the fertility potential improves. There are no definite guidelines; unprotected intercourse for a period of 1 year post-transplant is advised. Partner factor evaluation and assisted reproduction are the way forward in case of infertility. Data regarding the rationale of intrauterine insemination for male subfertility is debatable.[57] In vitro fertilization and ICSI are options in case of poor sperm parameters or female factor infertility or both. Surgical sperm retrieval may be required for men with azoospermia. Counseling should be done by a multidisciplinary team involving an andrologist, gynecologist, and an embryologist.

CONCLUSION

With improvements in treatment outcomes and survival after solid organ transplants, the prevalence of male SD and infertility continues to increase. The knowledge about these disturbances, etiology, and management strategies and prevention are essential to provide wholistic care to patients. These additional treatment tenets can improve long-term outcomes of men undergoing treatments such as transplant. Further, men undergoing treatment for hematopoietic diseases will benefit from fertility preservation, especially adolescents and young adults. Literature concerning liver, heart, and lung transplants are not yet robust and require more detailed documentation and assessment at a multicenter level.

KEY LEARNING POINTS

- Knowledge about changes in sperm parameters due to the basic disease such as CKD is important.
- Evaluation of sperm parameters prior to and after renal transplantation can guide in the treatment of male infertility.
- Immunosuppression may lead to sperm abnormalities, and it is wise to tailor the drugs based on the fertility status of the couple.
- Hormonal changes improve after renal transplant but may persist in some patients even after renal transplant.
- Pretransplant and preconceptional counseling play a valuable role in the treatment of male infertility.
- Fertility preservation is of paramount importance in men undergoing treatment of hematopoietic disorders which would damage spermatogenesis.

REFERENCES

1. Lundy SD, Vij SC. Male infertility in renal failure and transplantation. Transl Androl Urol. 2019;8(2):173-81.
2. Hart A, Smith JM, Skeans MA, Gustafson SK, Wilk AR, Robinson A, et al. OPTN/SRTR 2016 annual data report: kidney. Am J Transplant. 2018;18(Suppl. 1):18-113.
3. Agarwal A, Mulgund A, Hamada A, Chyatte MR. A unique view on male infertility around the globe. Reprod Biol Endocrinol. 2015;13:37.
4. Reinhardt W, Kübber H, Dolff S, Benson S, Führer D, Tan S. Rapid recovery of hypogonadism in male patients with end stage renal disease after renal transplantation. Endocrine. 2018;60(1):159-66.
5. Carrero JJ, Qureshi AR, Nakashima A, Arver S, Parini P, Lindholm B, et al. Prevalence and clinical implications of testosterone deficiency in men with end-stage renal disease. Nephrol Dial Transplant. 2011;26(1):184-90.
6. Akbari F, Alavi M, Esteghamati A, Mehrsai A, Djaladat H, Zohrevand R, et al. Effect of renal transplantation on sperm quality and sex hormone levels. BJU Int. 2003;92(3):281-3.
7. Wang GC, Zheng JH, Xu LG, Min ZL, Zhu YH, Qi J, et al. Measurements of serum pituitary-gonadal hormones and investigation of sexual and reproductive functions in kidney transplant recipients. Int J Nephrol. 2010;2010:612126.
8. Holley JL, Schmidt RJ. Changes in fertility and hormone replacement therapy in kidney disease. Adv Chronic Kidney Dis. 2013;20(3):240-5.
9. Handelsman DJ, Dong Q. Hypothalamo-pituitary gonadal axis in chronic renal failure. Endocrinol Metab Clin North Am. 1993;22(1):145-61.
10. Dumanski SM, Ahmed SB. Fertility and reproductive care in chronic kidney disease. J Nephrol. 2019;32(1):39-50.
11. Dunkel L, Raivio T, Laine J, Holmberg C. Circulating luteinizing hormone receptor inhibitor(s) in boys with chronic renal failure. Kidney Int. 1997;51(3):777-84.
12. Mitchell R, Bauerfeld C, Schaefer F, Schärer K, Robertson WR. Less acidic forms of luteinizing hormone are associated with lower testosterone secretion in men on haemodialysis treatment. Clin Endocrinol (Oxf). 1994;41(1):65-73.
13. Lehtihet M, Hylander B. Semen quality in men with chronic kidney disease and its correlation with chronic kidney disease stages. Andrologia. 2015;47(10):1103-08.
14. Lessan-Pezeshki M, Ghazizadeh S. Sexual and reproductive function in end-stage renal disease and effect of kidney transplantation. Asian J Androl. 2008;10(3):441-6.
15. Holley JL. The hypothalamic-pituitary axis in men and women with chronic kidney disease. Adv Chronic Kidney Dis. 2004;11(4):337-41.
16. Shiraishi K, Shimabukuro T, Naito K. Effects of hemodialysis on testicular volume and oxidative stress in humans. J Urol. 2008;180(2):644-50.
17. Xu LG, Shi SF, Qi XP, Huang XF, Xu HM, Song QZ, et al. Morphological characteristics of spermatozoa before and after renal transplantation. Asian J Androl. 2005;7(1):81-5.
18. Xu HM, Li HG, Xu LG, Zhang JR, Chen WY, Shi QX. The decline of fertility in male uremic patients is correlated with low expression of the cystic fibrosis transmembrane conductance regulator protein (CFTR) in human sperm. Hum Reprod. 2012;27(2):340-8.

19. Luciano RL, Dahl NK. Extra-renal manifestations of autosomal dominant polycystic kidney disease (ADPKD): considerations for routine screening and management. Nephrol Dial Transplant. 2014;29(2):247-54.
20. Woodhouse CR, Reilly JM, Bahadur G. Sexual function and fertility in patients treated for posterior urethral valves. J Urol. 1989;142(2 Pt 2):586-605.
21. Mieusset R, Fauquet I, Chauveau D, Monteil L, Chassaing N, Daudin M, et al. The spectrum of renal involvement in male patients with infertility related to excretory-system abnormalities: phenotypes, genotypes, and genetic counseling. J Nephrol. 2017;30(2):211-8.
22. Eid MM, Abdel-Hamid IA, Sobh MA, el-Saied MA. Assessment of sperm motion characteristics in infertile renal transplant recipients using computerized analysis. Int J Androl. 1996;19(6):338-44.
23. Papadopoulou E, Varouktsi A, Lazaridis A, Boutari C, Doumas M. Erectile dysfunction in chronic kidney disease: From pathophysiology to management. World J Nephrol. 2015;4(3):379-87.
24. Shamsa A, Motavalli SM, Aghdam B. Erectile function in end-stage renal disease before and after renal transplantation. Transplant Proc. 2005;37(7):3087-9.
25. Georgiou GK, Dounousi E, Harissis HV. Calcineurin inhibitors and male fertility after renal transplantation - a review. Andrologia. 2016;48(5):483-90.
26. Tondolo V, Citterio F, Panocchia N, Nanni G, Castagneto M. Sirolimus impairs improvement of the gonadal function after renal transplantation. Am J Transplant. 2005;5(1):197.
27. Zuber J, Anglicheau D, Elie C, Bererhi L, Timsit MO, Mamzer-Bruneel MF, et al. Sirolimus may reduce fertility in male renal transplant recipients. Am J Transplant. 2008;8(7):1471-9.
28. Tainio J, Jahnukainen K, Nurmio M, Pakarinen M, Jalanko H, Jahnukainen T. Testicular function, semen quality, and fertility in young men after renal transplantation during childhood or adolescence. Transplantation. 2014;98(9):987-93.
29. Barry JM. Spermatic cord preservation in kidney transplantation. J Urol. 1982;127(6):1076-7.
30. Perez-Aytes A, Ledo A, Boso V, Sáenz P, Roma E, Poveda JL, et al. In utero exposure to mycophenolate mofetil: a characteristic phenotype? Am J Med Genet A. 2008;146A(1):1-7.
31. Xu LG, Yang YR, Wang HW, Qiu F, Peng WL, Xu HM, et al. Characteristics of male fertility after renal transplantation. Andrologia. 2011;43(3):203-7.
32. Zeyneloglu HB, Oktem M, Durak T. Male infertility after renal transplantation: achievement of pregnancy after intracytoplasmic sperm injection. Transplant Proc. 2005;37(7):3081-4.
33. Veys KR, D'Hauwers KW, van Dongen AJCM, Janssen MC, Besouw MTP, Goossens E, et al. First successful conception induced by a male cystinosis patient. JIMD Rep. 2018;38:1-6.
34. Balmori C, Guillén A, Montans J, Bronet F, García-Velasco JA. Successful ICSI in an azoospermic and kidney transplant man with type 1 primary hyperoxaluria and first histopathological testicular findings described in the literature. Andrologia. 2015;47(1):109-11.
35. Lim VS. Reproductive function in patients with renal insufficiency. Am J Kidney Dis. 1987;9(4):363-7.

36. van Eps C, Hawley C, Jeffries J, Johnson DW, Campbell S, Isbel N, et al. Changes in serum prolactin, sex hormones and thyroid function with alternate nightly nocturnal home haemodialysis. Nephrology (Carlton). 2012;17(1):42-7.
37. Martin-Malo A, Benito P, Castillo D, Espinosa M, Burdiel LG, Perez R, et al. Effect of clomiphene citrate on hormonal profile in male hemodialysis and kidney transplant patients. Nephron. 1993;63(4):390-4.
38. Huang SA, Lie JD. Phosphodiesterase-5 (PDE5) inhibitors in the management of erectile dysfunction. P T. 2013;38(7):407-19.
39. Suzuki E, Nishimatsu H, Oba S, Takahashi M, Homma Y. Chronic kidney disease and erectile dysfunction. World J Nephrol. 2014;3(4):220-9.
40. Bhasin S, Cunningham GR, Hayes FJ, Matsumoto AM, Snyder PJ, Swerdloff RS, et al. Testosterone therapy in men with androgen deficiency syndromes: an Endocrine Society clinical practice guideline. J Clin Endocrinol Metab. 2010;95(6):2536-59. [published correction appears in J Clin Endocrinol Metab. 2021;106(7):e2848]
41. Hawksworth DJ, Burnett AL. Nonalcoholic fatty liver disease, male sexual dysfunction, and infertility: common links, common problems. Sex Med Rev. 2020;8(2):274-85.
42. Hofny ER, Ali ME, Taha EA, Nafeh HM, Sayed DS, Abdel-Azeem HG, et al. Semen and hormonal parameters in men with chronic hepatitis C infection. Fertil Steril. 2011;95(8):2557-9.
43. La Vignera S, Condorelli RA, Vicari E, D'Agata R, Calogero AE. Sperm DNA damage in patients with chronic viral C hepatitis. Eur J Intern Med. 2012;23(1):e19-24.
44. Huang JM, Huang TH, Qiu HY, Fang XW, Zhuang TG, Liu HX, et al. Effects of hepatitis B virus infection on human sperm chromosomes. World J Gastroenterol. 2003;9(4):736-40.
45. Huyghe E, Kamar N, Wagner F, Capietto AH, El-Kahwaji L, Muscari F, et al. Erectile dysfunction in end-stage liver disease men. J Sex Med. 2009;6(5):1395-401.
46. Wang YJ, Wu JC, Lee SD, Tsai YT, Lo KJ. Gonadal dysfunction and changes in sex hormones in postnecrotic cirrhotic men: a matched study with alcoholic cirrhotic men. Hepatogastroenterology. 1991;38(6):531-4.
47. Madersbacher S, Grünberger T, Maier U. Andrological status before and after liver transplantation. J Urol. 1994;151(5):1251-4.
48. Thakur J, Rathi S, Grover S, Chopra M, Agrawal S, Taneja S, et al. Tadalafil, a phosphodiesterase-5 inhibitor, improves erectile dysfunction in patients with liver cirrhosis. J Clin Exp Hepatol. 2019;9(3):312-7.
49. Sinclair M, Grossmann M, Gow PJ, Angus PW. Testosterone in men with advanced liver disease: abnormalities and implications. J Gastroenterol Hepatol. 2015;30(2):244-51.
50. De Luca MN, Colone M, Gambioli R, Stringaro A, Unfer V. Oxidative stress and male fertility: role of antioxidants and inositols. Antioxidants (Basel). 2021;10(8):1283.
51. Thirumavalavan N, Scovell JM, Link RE, Lamb DJ, Lipshultz LI. Does solid organ transplantation affect male reproduction? Eur Urol Focus. 2018;4(3):307-10.
52. Phelan R, Im A, Hunter RL, Inamoto Y, Lupo-Stanghellini MT, Rovo A, et al. Male-specific late effects in adult hematopoietic cell transplantation recipients: a systematic review from the Late Effects and Quality of Life Working Committee of the Center for International Blood and Marrow Transplant Research and

Transplant Complications Working Party of the European Society of Blood and Marrow Transplantation. Transplant Cell Ther. 2022;28(6):335.e1-17.
53. Joshi S, Savani BN, Chow EJ, Gilleece MH, Halter J, Jacobsohn DA, et al. Clinical guide to fertility preservation in hematopoietic cell transplant recipients. Bone Marrow Transplant. 2014;49(4):477-84.
54. Balduzzi A, Dalle JH, Jahnukainen K, von Wolff M, Lucchini G, Ifversen M, et al. Fertility preservation issues in pediatric hematopoietic stem cell transplantation: practical approaches from the consensus of the Pediatric Diseases Working Party of the EBMT and the International BFM Study Group. Bone Marrow Transplant. 2017;52(10):1406-15.
55. Hart A, Lentine KL, Smith JM, Miller JM, Skeans MA, Prentice M, et al. OPTN/SRTR 2019 annual data report: kidney. Am J Transplant. 2021;21(Suppl. 2):21-137.
56. Kandaswamy R, Stock PG, Miller J, Skeans MA, White J, Wainright J, et al. OPTN/SRTR 2019 annual data report: pancreas [published correction appears in Am J Transplant 2022;22(4):1283]. Am J Transplant. 2021;21(Suppl. 2):138-207.
57. Bensdorp AJ, Tjon-Kon-Fat RI, Bossuyt PMM, Koks CAM, Oosterhuis GJE, Hoek A, et al. Prevention of multiple pregnancies in couples with unexplained or mild male subfertility: randomised controlled trial of in vitro fertilisation with single embryo transfer or in vitro fertilisation in modified natural cycle compared with intrauterine insemination with controlled ovarian hyperstimulation. BMJ. 2015;350:g7771.

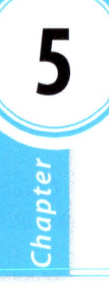

Chapter 5

Fertility and Assisted Reproductive Technology in Cancer Survivors: Breast Cancer

Kanad Dev Nayar, Ankita Sethi, Sakshi Miglani

■ INTRODUCTION

Breast malignancy is the most common malignancy in women worldwide.[1] During their lifetime, around 15% of women may have invasive breast cancer and around 6% in the age group <42 years. Literature shows that breast cancer is more aggressive and has unfavorable prognosis in younger women as compared to older women;[2] even though there has been a decline in the death rate,[3] still the 5-year survival rate in younger women (<40 years) is 85% as compared to almost 90% in older women.[4]

The inadequate disease awareness leads to worse prognosis in young women, and the features of breast cancer in reproductive age patients also vary with age at diagnosis.[4-8] Young patients (<40 years) may require chemotherapy, which have short-term and long-term adverse effects. Therefore, it is important for the treating clinicians to take into consideration the antagonistic effect of treatment on their quality of life.[9] Psychosocial issues are also common in these women that may influence their decision-making processes during care.[10] The cancer treatments have an adverse impact on fertility, which may decrease or eliminate childbearing potential in these women. There is an increasing trend of delaying childbearing.[11] Most women of reproductive age have not completed their family at the time of diagnosis, which makes treatment-related infertility as one of the most important problems.[12] Therefore, fertility preservation is the first step of management in these women before starting any gonadotoxic treatment.

It is crucial to discuss regarding the effect of chemotherapy and radiotherapy on ovarian reserve and future fertility with the patients. It is imperative that this should be part of multidisciplinary management of young breast cancer patients.[13] Despite clear recommendations by the European Society of Human Reproduction and Embryology (ESHRE) and other fertility societies on this, precancer treatment fertility preservation counseling is still underutilized.[4] In a survey done in young breast cancer patients between the ages of 20 and 45 years, <10% got any information or counseling regarding fertility preservation.[14] Other studies showed that these women were discontent with the information provided in terms of need of fertility preservation, and <15% were referred to a reproductive medicine specialist.[15]

Therefore, it is imperative for cancer specialists to counsel young breast cancer patients about fertility preservation and encourage a multidisciplinary approach toward their management.[4] According to several studies, the main concerns of these patients are the increased risk of cancer in offspring and risk of disease relapse and survivability. Majority patients were worried about treatment-associated infertility.[16,17] Research has shown that there is no difference in survival or recurrence after pregnancy in patients with completed treatment in either hormone receptor positive or negative breast cancer.[18]

In this chapter, we discuss the main treatment options that lead to ovarian dysfunction and various options of fertility preservation and the safety of pregnancy and breastfeeding after breast cancer.

FERTILITY PRESERVATION IN BREAST CANCER PATIENTS IN REPRODUCTIVE AGE GROUP

Oocyte Development (Oogenesis/Folliculogenesis)

Oogenesis is a process that starts during the embryonic stage; oogonia mature into the primary oocyte.[19] Primary oocytes are produced from oogonium during prenatal stage by mitosis. Primary oocyte enters the prophase of meiosis-I and gets arrested at this stage, until puberty. At puberty, under the influence of follicle-stimulating hormone (FSH) and luteinizing hormone (LH), the oocytes undergo maturation. The main role of FSH is in follicle selection and development.[20] Anti-Müllerian hormone (AMH) regulates follicular recruitment and reflects the follicle depletion. A recent study showed that AMH recovers by 18 months postchemotherapy to some extent but not completely.[21] Therefore, AMH may be used as an ovarian reserve marker in these patients undergoing chemotherapy or radiotherapy for prognostication.[16,22]

Treatment-induced Amenorrhea

Chemotherapy-induced amenorrhea means the cessation of menstruation postchemotherapy, which may or may not recover.[23] In 2020, Vriens et al. analyzed the ovarian function recovery rate at the end of 5 years post chemotherapy, which was around 90% and the 5-year live birth rate (LBR) post chemotherapy was 27% in breast cancer survivors.[24] Chemotherapy, hormone therapy, and different targeted agents have different gonadotoxic effects.

Chemotherapy

Different chemotherapeutic agents have different gonadotoxic effects, which are classified as high, intermediate, low, and unknown risk. Breast cancer patients undergoing chemotherapy at >40 years of age are at a greater risk of ovarian failure.[25] There are different LBR between cancer types, which is because of difference in the gonadotoxic effect of chemotherapeutic regimens.[24,26] The highest risk of premature ovarian failure is with alkylating agents, intermediate risk with anthracyclines and taxanes, and low risk with fluorouracil or methotrexate. Studies show that there is no difference in terms of gonadotoxicity between standard and dose-dense schedules.[27-30] Even though majority of women become amenorrheic during chemotherapy, almost 90% resume menstruation within 12 months of completion of treatment.[31]

Hormone Therapy

In patients with hormone receptor positive breast cancer, hormonal therapy is suggested for almost 10 years after diagnosis and completion of chemotherapy.

The various endocrine protocols available in premenopausal women for ovarian suppression are tamoxifen for 5 years and aromatase inhibitor (AI) for 5 years. The high-risk disease patients benefit maximum from these protocols, and there is little difference in efficacy between different protocols.[32,33] Tamoxifen may decrease the chances of pregnancy in breast cancer survivor patients as it changes the hormonal levels, which leads to menstrual irregularity or cessation of menstruation but does not cause direct ovarian damage. Tamoxifen inhibits the hypothalamic–pituitary–ovarian (HPO) axis, which leads to an increase in steroidogenesis in the ovary. Literature suggests that tamoxifen can lead to a decrease in AMH and rising FSH levels; therefore, tamoxifen is considered as an amenorrhea-inducing low-risk agent.[34] Pregnancy is contraindicated during hormonal therapy as it has teratogenic effects. By the time the adjuvant hormonal therapy ends, majority of women are either perimenopausal or even postmenopausal.[35]

Targeted Therapy

There is small data on the effect of immunotherapy, tyrosine kinase inhibitors, or antihuman epidermal growth factor receptor 2 (HER-2) agents on the reproductive system. One study showed that when trastuzumab was added to chemotherapy, it did not show any increase in treatment-induced amenorrhea.[36] Premenopausal breast cancer patients who received paclitaxel–trastuzumab combination in one of the trials had less therapy-related amenorrhea than earlier data on alkylating agents.[37] In a recent study by Ruddy et al. (2021), they took chemotherapy-related amenorrhea (CRA) as a surrogate for ovarian toxicity and associated risk of infertility and premature menopause. They compared CRA rate with paclitaxel (T)-trastuzumab (H) to that with ado-trastuzumab emtansine (T-DM1) and found that amenorrhea at 18 months was less likely in recipients of adjuvant T-DM1 (targeted therapy) than TH.[38]

Radiotherapy

The breast radiotherapy for breast cancer treatment has nominal effect on ovarian function, but fertility preservation and gestation should be avoided during radiotherapy.[39]

Fertility Preservation Strategies

In vitro fertilization (IVF) is defined as fertilization of oocytes and sperm in an embryology laboratory.[40] In a routine IVF cycle, numerous follicles in the ovary are stimulated to produce oocytes, thereby improving the cumulative LBR. This process is called controlled ovarian stimulation (COS) and is preferred over a single oocyte that is produced naturally.[41] Fertility preservation options in these breast cancer patients can be cryopreservation of embryos and/or oocytes.

Embryo/Oocyte Cryopreservation

The COS and embryo/oocyte vitrification are the treatment of choice for fertility preservation. Vitrification is the established process of fast freezing oocytes/embryos in liquid nitrogen at temperatures as low as −30,000°C. Either oocyte or embryo cryopreservation can be considered depending upon individual circumstances as both are well-established techniques for fertility preservation. Due to the age-related decrement in the number of antral follicles, fertility preservation has lower success rates at >40 years of age. As the age increases, the efficiency of the vitrified oocytes decreases from 7.4% at age 30 years to 5.2% for more than 38 years.[42]

Ovarian Tissue Cryopreservation and Reimplantation

Before the commencement of chemotherapy, either a part of or the whole ovary is surgically removed, and ovarian cortex is cryopreserved, which allows the reimplantation whenever desired. According to the various guidelines and recommendations, it is still considered an experimental technique.[1,28] The main advantage is that ovarian stimulation is not required, which prevents any treatment delay. It preserves both fertility and gonadal function, and the patient can try natural conception also.[43] However, ovarian tissue cryopreservation (OTC) and reimplantation will require two surgical procedures, which can lead to an increased risk of ischemia to the follicle. There is also a risk of malignant contamination/reseeding malignant cells at the time of reimplantation. OTC is not considered for *BRCA* carriers, both because of the associated risk of ovarian cancer and risk of reimplanting malignant cells.[44] OTC is the treatment of choice in prepubertal girls and in women where treatment delay is not possible like in advanced breast cancer where immediate treatment initiation is required, and in patients at high risk of premature ovarian failure.[45]

In Vitro Maturation

Clinical definition of IVM is the aspiration of small or intermediate-sized follicles for oocyte retrieval in the ovaries carrying follicles less than 13 mm in diameter. Short-course of gonadotropin is given which leads to retrieval of immature oocytes. This offers better flexibility, less drugs are required for ovarian stimulation, there is minimum exposure to raised estradiol levels, and the cost of ovarian stimulation decreases.[46] The disadvantage is the low success rate as compared to conventional fertility preservation techniques.[47,48] Even though it is used mainly in research settings, it is feasible for patients who want oocyte or embryo vitrification but cannot delay chemotherapy.[49] Studies have shown that assisted reproductive technology (ART) success rates in patients with cancer are similar to their age-specified general population.[40]

Ovarian Suppression During Chemotherapy

Transient ovarian suppression, which is attained pharmacologically, aims to prevent gonadotoxicity induced by chemotherapy, with the principal aim of decreasing the risk of premature ovarian failure. Literature shows that transient ovarian suppression with gonadotropin-releasing hormone agonist (GnRHa) is safe and efficacious, and their main role is to decrease the mitosis in granulosa cells of the ovary.[50] Lambertini et al. in their meta-analysis suggested that the usage of GnRHa during chemotherapy in reproductive age group breast cancer patients could reduce premature ovarian failure and improve pregnancy rates.[51] Still, there is no agreement on the usage of GnRHa during chemotherapy in reproductive age group patients; further research and follow-up studies are required. However, the transient ovarian suppression option can be given to women not keen for further pregnancies, for preserving the ovarian function in women aged 40–45 years, or in patients who underwent fertility preservation with embryo vitrification. They should also use GnRHa to preserve the gonadal function.[28,52,53]

Controlled Ovarian Stimulation

A COS cycle delays the chemotherapy by at least 2 weeks [average 12 days (10–19 days)].[46] Patients with breast cancer generally have an interval of 4–6 weeks between surgical procedure and chemotherapy.[54] This time duration is adequate to carry out COS without delaying the start of chemotherapy. Nevertheless, patients who require neoadjuvant chemotherapy may have less time between diagnosis and treatment initiation. The literature and recommendations highlight the importance of early referrals for fertility preservation.

The patients who received neoadjuvant chemotherapy had lower fertility preservation rate as compared to patients with primary surgical management.[55]

Generally, there are three types of COS protocols: GnRHa short or long protocols, GnRH antagonists, or GnRH antagonists plus letrozole for hormone-dependent tumors. But in breast cancer patients where chemotherapy has to be started as early as possible, long GnRHa protocols are not used; therefore random start GnRH antagonist protocols (with or without letrozole) are used for fertility preservation. One more drawback of GnRHa protocols is the enhanced risk of ovarian hyperstimulation syndrome (OHSS).[56] In GnRH antagonist protocols, GnRHa trigger is used, which decreases the estradiol levels after oocyte retrieval, therefore reducing OHSS risk.[56] Wang et al. conducted a meta-analysis, compared GnRH antagonist and agonist protocols, and included almost 30 randomized controlled trials (RCTs) and almost 6,400 women.[57] There was not much difference in terms of LBR, and the GnRH antagonist protocol has the advantage of random start in the follicular or luteal phase.[58] Nowadays, all ovarian stimulation protocols used in fertility preservation use AIs to suppress the estradiol levels, especially in hormone-dependent tumors.[59] Studies show no increased risk of recurrence when letrozole is added to the stimulation protocols.[60]

A study showed no difference in survival of patients who underwent letrozole-based COS versus no stimulation.[61] Literature shows that letrozole is better than tamoxifen for this purpose.[62]

Long-term Safety of COS in Breast Cancer Patients and Preconceptional Counseling

Since breast malignancies are hormone dependent, both the patients in their reproductive age group and their treating physicians are concerned about the safety of fertility preservation techniques. This is because of the limited literature on long-term safety of fertility preservation including ovarian stimulation in breast cancer patients. A recent meta-analysis showed that there is no harmful effect of COS with similar results in all the studies. Another meta-analysis[63] reported that use of letrozole decreases the serum estradiol levels and it does not affect the COS outcomes. Hence, letrozole inclusion in the COS protocol is now standard in all COS, especially if it is hormone positive in breast cancer patients.

A recent meta-analysis also reported that there are only two studies that that address the survival outcomes as per the hormone receptor status of the tumor; no detrimental effect of ovarian stimulation on survival was found. The Pregnancy and Fertility (PREFER) meta-analysis study[64] showed that almost 10% of the reproductive age group breast cancer patients refuse fertility preservation with the fear of delay in chemotherapy.

Since breast cancer is not as aggressive as compared to the aggressive hematological cancer, a short time duration, that is, 7–10 days, should not be considered as a contraindication to fertility preservation for the majority of patients. It has been seen that adjuvant chemotherapy is effective up to

12 weeks after surgery, even though maximum time should be maximum 60 days, especially for patients with aggressive cancer at a greater risk of relapse such as triple-negative or HER2 positive cancer.[65,66] This can be applicable for neoadjuvant chemotherapy as well.[67] According to literature, the average time from diagnosis to initiation of chemotherapy is 35–45 days.[68] Therefore, a delay of 6 days should not be clinically significant and would not exceed the maximum 60 day. Research shows that there is no increased recurrence risk after COS for fertility preservation in the reproductive age group breast cancer patients.[69]

Very limited data is available on the safety of COS in breast cancer survivors after chemotherapy completion.[70-72] Only four studies are there on COS after chemotherapy in breast cancer survivors, which have shown that there is no increased recurrence risk and no increased chance of empty follicle syndrome.[71]

■ PREGNANCY AND BREAST CANCER SURVIVAL OUTCOMES

A meta-analysis reported that pregnancy after breast cancer was associated with a reduced fatality rate [hazard ratio (HR): 0.6].[73] Lambertini reported no difference between hormone receptor positive patients who became pregnant and those who did not in terms of disease free survival or overall survival.[74] There is no conclusive data on the ideal time for pregnancy after breast cancer diagnosis and treatment. However, the recommendation proposes that a patient should wait for at least 2 years after diagnosis and treatment for the ovarian function to recover, and the recurrence risk is minimized.[75] After hormonal therapy, patients should wait for at least 2–3 months for complete washout before trying for pregnancy.[76] Majority of the studies are retrospective, and prospective data is required.

Effect on Pregnancy Outcome

Studies show a relatively high miscarriage rate (21–43%) in breast cancer survivors.[77-83] This data shows the uncertainties and anxiety faced by breast cancer survivors and their oncologists about the safety of pregnancy post-treatment.

Recent large cohort studies on breast cancer survivors and pregnancy have some reassuring results,[84,85] even though Dalberg et al. *found an increased risk of* cesarean section, preterm birth, and low birth weight in breast cancer survivors.[84] Hence, breast cancer survivors who become pregnant should be considered high-risk pregnancy and should be followed in a tertiary care center with good obstetrics and neonatal intensive care unit (NICU) facility.

■ BREASTFEEDING IN BREAST CANCER SURVIVORS

Breastfeeding is related to the overall reduced lifetime risk of breast cancer.[86,87] Therefore, the World Health Organization (WHO) initiatives propose to improve breastfeeding rates worldwide. There is lack of data on breastfeeding-related problems of breast cancer patients after treatment. In patients undergoing conservative surgery, one of the main concerns is the ability to breastfeed from the affected breast. In majority of cases where the breast has undergone radiotherapy, there are irreversible fibrosis and vascular changes.[88] Therefore, women should be reassured that they can breastfeed from untreated breast, can produce sufficient milk, and can feed from unilateral breast.[89] They should lactate only from the unaffected breast.[90] Lactation is contraindicated during neoadjuvant chemotherapy (NACT) as it has longer $t_{1/2}$ and a higher excretion rate in breastmilk.[91] Limited data is available for monoclonal antibodies. Hormonal therapy is detected and accumulates in breastmilk over time and therefore is contraindicated during breastfeeding. Women with hormone receptor-positive breast cancer should complete a minimum of 18-24 months of hormonal therapy before considering pregnancy or breastfeeding.[53]

■ CONCLUSION

For the last few years, there has been an increase in the diagnosis of breast cancer in reproductive age women, along with better detection and management, which result in better survival. In these reproductive age women diagnosed with breast cancer, it is imperative for the oncologist to assess the desire for fertility preservation. Fertility preservation options should be individualized. Even though there is limited data, pregnancy is safe after chemotherapy and radiotherapy. There are many ongoing studies which will give data on pregnancy safety and outcomes, and accordingly, these women can be counseled regarding fertility preservation, pregnancy, and breastfeeding.

KEY LEARNING POINTS

- During their lifetime, around 15% of women may have invasive breast cancer and around 6% in the age group <42 years.
- There has been an increase in the diagnosis of breast cancer in reproductive age women, along with better detection and management, which result in better survival. Thus, fertility preservation counseling and techniques are utmost important for these patients. They should receive multidisciplinary management.
- Despite clear recommendations by ESHRE and other fertility societies on this, precancer treatment fertility preservation counseling is still underutilized.
- Fertility preservation options should be individualized such as oocyte or embryo cryopreservation or OTC.
- Literature suggests that there is no harmful effect of COS and no increased recurrence risk either when COS is done before chemotherapy or after completion of treatment, that is, in breast cancer survivors.

■ REFERENCES

1. Cardoso F, Kyriakides S, Ohno S, Penault-Llorca F, Poortmans P, Rubio IT, et al. Early breast cancer: ESMO Clinical Practice Guidelines for diagnosis, treatment and follow-up. Ann Oncol. 2019;30(8):1194-220.
2. Anders CK, Johnson R, Litton J, Phillips M, Bleyer A. Breast cancer before age 40 years. Semin Oncol. 2009;36(3):237-49.
3. DeSantis CE, Ma J, Gaudet MM, Newman LA, Miller KD, Goding Sauer A, et al. Breast cancer statistics, 2019. CA Cancer J Clin. 2019;69(6):438-51.
4. Martinez F, Andersen CY, Barri PN, Brannigan R, Cobo A, Donnez J, et al. Update on fertility preservation from the Barcelona International Society for Fertility Preservation-ESHRE-ASRM 2015 expert meeting: indications, results and future perspectives. Fertil Steril. 2017;108(3):407-15.e11.
5. Azim HA, Michiels S, Bedard PL, Singhal SK, Criscitiello C, Ignatiadis M, et al. Elucidating prognosis and biology of breast cancer arising in young women using gene expression profiling. Clin Cancer Res. 2012;18(5):1341-51.
6. Collins LC, Marotti JD, Gelber S, Cole K, Ruddy K, Kereakoglow S, et al. Pathologic features and molecular phenotype by patient age in a large cohort of young women with breast cancer. Breast Cancer Res Treat. 2012;131(3):1061-6.
7. Keegan THM, DeRouen MC, Press DJ, Kurian AW, Clarke CA. Occurrence of breast cancer subtypes in adolescent and young adult women. Breast Cancer Res. 2012;14(2):R55.
8. Oltra SS, Peña-Chilet M, Vidal-Tomas V, Flower K, Martinez MT, Alonso E, et al. Methylation deregulation of miRNA promoters identifies miR124-2 as a survival biomarker in breast cancer in very young women. Sci Rep. 2018;8(1):14373.
9. Francis PA, Regan MM, Fleming GF, Láng I, Ciruelos E, Bellet M, et al. Adjuvant ovarian suppression in premenopausal breast cancer. N Engl J Med. 2015;372(5):436-46.
10. Llarena NC, Estevez SL, Tucker SL, Jeruss JS. Impact of fertility concerns on tamoxifen initiation and persistence. J Natl Cancer Inst. 2015;107(10):djv202.
11. Matthews TJ, Hamilton BE. First births to older women continue to rise. NCHS Data Brief. 2014;(152):1-8.
12. Cooke A, Mills TA, Lavender T. 'Informed and uninformed decision making'— Women's reasoning, experiences and perceptions with regard to advanced maternal age and delayed childbearing: a meta-synthesis. Int J Nurs Stud. 2010;47(10):1317-29.
13. Lambertini M, Goldrat O, Ferreira AR, Dechene J, Azim HA, Desir J, et al. Reproductive potential and performance of fertility preservation strategies in BRCA-mutated breast cancer patients. Ann Oncol. 2018;29(1):237-43.
14. Goldfarb SB, Kamer SA, Oppong BA, Eaton A, Patil S, Junqueira MJ, et al. Fertility preservation in the young breast cancer patient. Ann Surg Oncol. 2016;23(5):1530-6.
15. Scanlon M, Blaes A, Geller M, Majhail NS, Lindgren B, Haddad T. Patient satisfaction with physician discussions of treatment impact on fertility, menopause and sexual health among pre-menopausal women with cancer. J Cancer. 2012;3:217-25.
16. Ruddy KJ, Gelber SI, Tamimi RM, Ginsburg ES, Schapira L, Come SE, et al. Prospective study of fertility concerns and preservation strategies in young women with breast cancer. J Clin Oncol. 2014;32(11):1151-6.

17. Ruggeri M, Pagan E, Bagnardi V, Bianco N, Gallerani E, Buser K, et al. Fertility concerns, preservation strategies and quality of life in young women with breast cancer: baseline results from an ongoing prospective cohort study in selected European centers. Breast. 2019;47:85-92.
18. Azim HA, Kroman N, Paesmans M, Gelber S, Rotmensz N, Ameye L, et al. Prognostic impact of pregnancy after breast cancer according to estrogen receptor status: a multicenter retrospective study. J Clin Oncol. 2013;31(1):73-9.
19. Johnson J, Canning J, Kaneko T, Pru JK, Tilly JL. Germline stem cells and follicular renewal in the postnatal mammalian ovary. Nature. 2004;428(6979):145-50.
20. Jaffe LA, Egbert JR. Regulation of mammalian oocyte meiosis by intercellular communication within the ovarian follicle. Annu Rev Physiol. 2017;79(1):237-60.
21. Goldfarb SB, Turan V, Bedoschi G, Taylan E, Abdo N, Cigler T, et al. Impact of adjuvant chemotherapy or tamoxifen-alone on the ovarian reserve of young women with breast cancer. Breast Cancer Res Treat. 2021;185(1):165-73. doi: 10.1007/s10549-020-05933-7. Epub 2020 Sep 15. PMID: 32930927; PMCID: PMC7877450.
22. Bozza C, Puglisi F, Lambertini M, Osa EO, Manno M, Del Mastro L. Anti-Müllerian hormone: determination of ovarian reserve in early breast cancer patients. Endocr Relat Cancer. 2014;21(1):R51-65.
23. Liedtke C, Kiesel L. Chemotherapy-induced amenorrhea – an update. Geburtsh Frauenheilk. 2012;72(09):809-18.
24. Vriens IJH, De Bie AJR, Aarts MJB, de Boer M, van Hellemond IEG, Roijen JHE, et al. The correlation of age with chemotherapy-induced ovarian function failure in breast cancer patients. Oncotarget. 2017;8(7):11372-9.
25. Beck-Peccoz P, Persani L. Premature ovarian failure. Orphanet J Rare Dis. 2006;1(1):9.
26. Petrek JA, Naughton MJ, Case LD, Paskett ED, Naftalis EZ, Singletary SE, et al. Incidence, time course, and determinants of menstrual bleeding after breast cancer treatment: a prospective study. J Clin Oncol. 2006;24(7):1045-51.
27. Lambertini M, Ceppi M, Cognetti F, Cavazzini G, De Laurentiis M, De Placido S, et al. Dose-dense adjuvant chemotherapy in premenopausal breast cancer patients: a pooled analysis of the MIG1 and GIM2 phase III studies. Eur J Cancer. 2017;71:34-42.
28. Oktay K, Harvey BE, Partridge AH, Quinn GP, Reinecke J, Taylor HS, et al. Fertility preservation in patients with cancer: ASCO clinical practice guideline update. J Clin Oncol. 2018;36(19):1994-2001.
29. Pérez-Fidalgo JA, Roselló S, García-Garré E, Jordá E, Martín-Martorell P, Bermejo B, et al. Incidence of chemotherapy-induced amenorrhea in hormone-sensitive breast cancer patients: the impact of addition of taxanes to anthracycline-based regimens. Breast Cancer Res Treat. 2010;120(1):245-51.
30. Tomasi-Cont N, Lambertini M, Hulsbosch S, Peccatori AF, Amant F. Strategies for fertility preservation in young early breast cancer patients. Breast. 2014;23(5):503-10.
31. Waks AG, Partridge AH. Fertility preservation in patients with breast cancer: necessity, methods, and safety. J Natl Compr Canc Netw. 2016;14(3):355-63.
32. Davies C, Pan H, Godwin J, Gray R, Arriagada R, Raina V, et al. Long-term effects of continuing adjuvant tamoxifen to 10 years versus stopping at 5 years after diagnosis of oestrogen receptor-positive breast cancer: ATLAS, a randomised trial. Lancet. 2013;381(9869):805-16.

33. Francis PA, Pagani O, Fleming GF, Walley BA, Colleoni M, Láng I, et al. Tailoring adjuvant endocrine therapy for premenopausal breast cancer. N Engl J Med. 2018;379(2):122-37.
34. Partridge AH, Ruddy KJ, Gelber S, Schapira L, Abusief M, Meyer M, et al. Ovarian reserve in women who remain premenopausal after chemotherapy for early stage breast cancer. Fertil Steril. 2010;94(2):638-44.
35. McCray DKS, Simpson AB, Flyckt R, Liu Y, O'Rourke C, Crowe JP, et al. Fertility in women of reproductive age after breast cancer treatment: practice patterns and outcomes. Ann Surg Oncol. 2016;23(10):3175-81.
36. Abusief ME, Missmer SA, Ginsburg ES, Weeks JC, Partridge AH. The effects of paclitaxel, dose density, and trastuzumab on treatment-related amenorrhea in premenopausal women with breast cancer. Cancer. 2010;116(4):791-8.
37. Ruddy KJ, Guo H, Barry W, Dang CT, Yardley DA, Moy B, et al. Chemotherapy-related amenorrhea after adjuvant paclitaxel–trastuzumab (APT trial). Breast Cancer Res Treat. 2015;151(3):589-96.
38. Ruddy KJ, Zheng Y, Tayob N, Hu J, Dang CT, Yardley DA, et al. Chemotherapy-related amenorrhea (CRA) after adjuvant ado-trastuzumab emtansine (T-DM1) compared to paclitaxel in combination with trastuzumab (TH) (TBCRC033: ATEMPT Trial). Breast Cancer Res Treat. 2021;189(1):103-10.
39. Gonçalves V, Quinn GP. Review of fertility preservation issues for young women with breast cancer. Hum Fertil. 2016;19(3):152-65.
40. Carneiro MM, Cota AM, Amaral MC, Pedrosa ML, Martins BO, Furtado MH, et al. Motherhood after breast cancer: can we balance fertility preservation and cancer treatment? A narrative review of the literature. JBRA Assist Reprod. 2018;22(3):244-52.
41. Dolmans MM, Lambertini M, Macklon KT, Almeida Santos T, Ruiz-Casado A, Borini A, et al. EUropean REcommendations for female FERtility preservation (EU-REFER): a joint collaboration between oncologists and fertility specialists. Crit Rev Oncol Hematol. 2019;138:233-40.
42. Doyle JO, Richter KS, Lim J, Stillman RJ, Graham JR, Tucker MJ. Successful elective and medically indicated oocyte vitrification and warming for autologous in vitro fertilization, with predicted birth probabilities for fertility preservation according to number of cryopreserved oocytes and age at retrieval. Fertil Steril. 2016;105(2):459-66.e2.
43. Donnez J, Dolmans MM. Ovarian cortex transplantation: 60 reported live births brings the success and worldwide expansion of the technique towards routine clinical practice. J Assist Reprod Genet. 2015;32(8):1167-70.
44. Kasum M, von Wolff M, Franulić D, Čehić E, Klepac-Pulanić T, Orešković S, et al. Fertility preservation options in breast cancer patients. Gynecol Endocrinol. 2015;31(11):846-51.
45. Diaz-Garcia C, Domingo J, Garcia-Velasco JA, Herraiz S, Mirabet V, Iniesta I, et al. Oocyte vitrification versus ovarian cortex transplantation in fertility preservation for adult women undergoing gonadotoxic treatments: a prospective cohort study. Fertil Steril. 2018;109(3):478-85.e2.
46. Reddy J, Oktay K. Ovarian stimulation and fertility preservation with the use of aromatase inhibitors in women with breast cancer. Fertil Steril. 2012;98(6):1363-9.
47. De Pedro M, Otero B, Martín B. Fertility preservation and breast cancer: a review. ecancer. 2015;9.

48. Levine JM, Kelvin JF, Quinn GP, Gracia CR. Infertility in reproductive-age female cancer survivors: infertility in female cancer survivors. Cancer. 2015;121(10):1532-9.
49. Chian RC, Uzelac PS, Nargund G. In vitro maturation of human immature oocytes for fertility preservation. Fertil Steril. 2013;99(5):1173-81.
50. Elgindy EA. Progesterone level and progesterone/estradiol ratio on the day of hCG administration: detrimental cutoff levels and new treatment strategy. Fertil Steril. 2011;95(5):1639-44.
51. Lambertini M, Moore HCF, Leonard RCF, Loibl S, Munster P, Bruzzone M, et al. Gonadotropin-releasing hormone agonists during chemotherapy for preservation of ovarian function and fertility in premenopausal patients with early breast cancer: a systematic review and meta-analysis of individual patient-level data. J Clin Oncol. 2018;36(19):1981-90.
52. Lambertini M, Cinquini M, Moschetti I, Peccatori FA, Anserini P, Valenzano Menada M, et al. Temporary ovarian suppression during chemotherapy to preserve ovarian function and fertility in breast cancer patients: a GRADE approach for evidence evaluation and recommendations by the Italian Association of Medical Oncology. Eur J Cancer. 2017;71:25-33.
53. Paluch-Shimon S, Cardoso F, Partridge AH, Abulkhair O, Azim HA, Bianchi-Micheli G, et al. ESO–ESMO 4th International Consensus Guidelines for Breast Cancer in Young Women (BCY4). Ann Oncol. 2020;31(6):674-96.
54. Turan V, Bedoschi G, Moy F, Oktay K. Safety and feasibility of performing two consecutive ovarian stimulation cycles with the use of letrozole-gonadotropin protocol for fertility preservation in breast cancer patients. Fertil Steril. 2013;100(6):1681-5.e1.
55. Constance ES, Moravek MB, Jeruss JS. Strategies to maintain fertility in young breast cancer patients. In: Gradishar WJ (Ed). Optimizing Breast Cancer Management [Internet]. Cham: Springer International Publishing; 2018. pp. 1-13.
56. Humaidan P, Quartarolo J, Papanikolaou EG. Preventing ovarian hyperstimulation syndrome: guidance for the clinician. Fertil Steril. 2010;94(2):389-400.
57. Wang R, Lin S, Wang Y, Qian W, Zhou L. Comparisons of GnRH antagonist protocol versus GnRH agonist long protocol in patients with normal ovarian reserve: a systematic review and meta-analysis. PLoS One. 2017;12(4):e0175985.
58. Sönmezer M, Türkçüoğlu I, Coşkun U, Oktay K. Random-start controlled ovarian hyperstimulation for emergency fertility preservation in letrozole cycles. Fertil Steril. 2011;95(6):2125.e9-11.
59. Bedoschi G, Oktay K. Current approach to fertility preservation by embryo cryopreservation. Fertil Steril. 2013;99(6):1496-502.
60. Kim SS. Assessment of long term endocrine function after transplantation of frozen-thawed human ovarian tissue to the heterotopic site: 10 year longitudinal follow-up study. J Assist Reprod Genet. 2012;29(6):489-93.
61. Kim J, Turan V, Oktay K. Long-term safety of letrozole and gonadotropin stimulation for fertility preservation in women with breast cancer. J Clin Endocrinol Metab. 2016;101(4):1364-71.
62. Oktay K, Buyuk E, Libertella N, Akar M, Rosenwaks Z. Fertility preservation in breast cancer patients: a prospective controlled comparison of ovarian stimulation with tamoxifen and letrozole for embryo cryopreservation. J Clin Oncol. 2005;23(19):4347-53.

63. Bonardi B, Massarotti C, Bruzzone M, Goldrat O, Mangili G, Anserini P, et al. Efficacy and safety of controlled ovarian stimulation with or without letrozole co-administration for fertility preservation: a systematic review and meta-analysis. Front Oncol. 2020;10:574669.
64. Blondeaux E, Massarotti C, Fontana V, Poggio F, Arecco L, Fregatti P, et al. The PREgnancy and FERtility (PREFER) study investigating the need for ovarian function and/or fertility preservation strategies in premenopausal women with early breast cancer. Front Oncol. 2021;11:690320.
65. Lohrisch C, Paltiel C, Gelmon K, Speers C, Taylor S, Barnett J, et al. Impact on survival of time from definitive surgery to initiation of adjuvant chemotherapy for early-stage breast cancer. J Clin Oncol. 2006;24(30):4888-94.
66. de Melo Gagliato D, Gonzalez-Angulo AM, Lei X, Theriault RL, Giordano SH, Valero V, et al. Clinical impact of delaying initiation of adjuvant chemotherapy in patients with breast cancer. J Clin Oncol. 2014;32(8):735-44.
67. de Melo Gagliato D, Lei X, Giordano SH, Valero V, Barcenas CH, Hortobagyi GN, et al. Impact of delayed neoadjuvant systemic chemotherapy on overall survival among patients with breast cancer. Oncologist. 2020;25(9):749-57.
68. Moravek MB, Confino R, Lawson AK, Smith KN, Kazer RR, Klock SC, et al. Predictors and outcomes in breast cancer patients who did or did not pursue fertility preservation. Breast Cancer Res Treat. 2021;186(2):429-37.
69. Lambertini M, Peccatori FA, Demeestere I, Amant F, Wyns C, Stukenborg JB, et al. Fertility preservation and post-treatment pregnancies in post-pubertal cancer patients: ESMO clinical practice guidelines. Ann Oncol. 2020;31(12):1664-78.
70. Goldrat O, Kroman N, Peccatori FA, Cordoba O, Pistilli B, Lidegaard O, et al. Pregnancy following breast cancer using assisted reproduction and its effect on long-term outcome. Eur J Cancer. 2015;51(12):1490-6.
71. Rosenberg E, Fredriksson A, Einbeigi Z, Bergh C, Strandell A. No increased risk of relapse of breast cancer for women who give birth after assisted conception. Hum Reprod Open. 2019;2019(4):hoz039.
72. Condorelli M, Bruzzone M, Ceppi M, Ferrari A, Grinshpun A, Hamy AS, et al. Safety of assisted reproductive techniques in young women harboring germline pathogenic variants in BRCA1/2 with a pregnancy after prior history of breast cancer. ESMO Open. 2021;6(6):100300.
73. Hartman EK, Eslick GD. The prognosis of women diagnosed with breast cancer before, during and after pregnancy: a meta-analysis. Breast Cancer Res Treat. 2016;160(2):347-60.
74. Lambertini M, Goldrat O, Clatot F, Demeestere I, Awada A. Controversies about fertility and pregnancy issues in young breast cancer patients: current state of the art. Curr Opin Oncol. 2017;29(4):243-52.
75. Cardoso F, Loibl S, Pagani O, Graziottin A, Panizza P, Martincich L, et al. The European Society of Breast Cancer Specialists recommendations for the management of young women with breast cancer. Eur J Cancer. 2012;48(18):3355-77.
76. Braems G, Denys H, De Wever O, Cocquyt V, Van den Broecke R. Use of tamoxifen before and during pregnancy. Oncologist. 2011;16(11):1547-51.
77. Ives A, Saunders C, Bulsara M, Semmens J. Pregnancy after breast cancer: population based study. BMJ. 2007;334(7586):194.

78. Kroman N, Jensen MB, Melbye M, Wohlfahrt J, Mouridsen HT. Should women be advised against pregnancy after breast-cancer treatment? Lancet. 1997;350(9074):319-22.
79. Velentgas P, Daling JR, Malone KE, Weiss NS, Williams MA, Self SG, et al. Pregnancy after breast carcinoma: outcomes and influence on mortality. Cancer. 1999;85(11):2424-32.
80. Gelber S, Coates AS, Goldhirsch A, Castiglione-Gertsch M, Marini G, Lindtner J, et al. Effect of pregnancy on overall survival after the diagnosis of early-stage breast cancer. J Clin Oncol. 2001;19(6):1671-5.
81. Lawrenz B, Henes M, Neunhoeffer E, Fehm T, Huebner S, Kanz L, et al. Pregnancy after successful cancer treatment: what needs to be considered? Onkologie. 2012;35(3):128-32.
82. Córdoba O, Bellet M, Vidal X, Cortés J, Llurba E, Rubio IT, et al. Pregnancy after treatment of breast cancer in young women does not adversely affect the prognosis. Breast. 2012;21(3):272-5.
83. von Schoultz E, Johansson H, Wilking N, Rutqvist LE. Influence of prior and subsequent pregnancy on breast cancer prognosis. J Clin Oncol. 1995;13(2):430-4.
84. Dalberg K, Eriksson J, Holmberg L. Birth outcome in women with previously treated breast cancer—a population-based cohort study from Sweden. PLoS Med. 2006;3(9):e336.
85. Langagergaard V, Gislum M, Skriver MV, Nørgård B, Lash TL, Rothman KJ, et al. Birth outcome in women with breast cancer. Br J Cancer. 2006;94(1):142-6.
86. Anothaisintawee T, Wiratkapun C, Lerdsitthichai P, Kasamesup V, Wongwaisayawan S, Srinakarin J, et al. Risk factors of breast cancer: a systematic review and meta-analysis. Asia Pac J Public Health. 2013;25(5):368-87.
87. Freund C, Mirabel L, Annane K, Mathelin C. Allaitement maternel et cancer du sein. Gynécol Obstét Fertil. 2005;33(10):739-44.
88. Moore GH, Schiller JE, Moore GK. Radiation-induced histopathologic changes of the breast: the effects of time. Am J Surg Pathol. 2004;28(1):47-53.
89. Michaels AM, Wanner H. Breastfeeding twins after mastectomy. J Hum Lact. 2013;29(1):20-2.
90. Shachar SS, Gallagher K, McGuire K, Zagar TM, Faso A, Muss HB, et al. Multidisciplinary management of breast cancer during pregnancy. Oncologist. 2017;22(3):324-34.
91. Pistilli B, Bellettini G, Giovannetti E, Codacci-Pisanelli G, Azim HA, Benedetti G, et al. Chemotherapy, targeted agents, antiemetics and growth-factors in human milk: how should we counsel cancer patients about breastfeeding? Cancer Treat Rev. 2013;39(3):207-11.

Fertility and Assisted Reproductive Technology in Cancer Survivors: Endometrial Cancer

Surveen Ghumman Sindhu

■ INTRODUCTION

Endometrial cancer is an important malignancy. The most important aspect of the disease is cure and rehabilitation. Cure requires surgical removal of lesion, chemotherapy, and radiotherapy. Chemotherapy and radiotherapy may impair fertility in varying degrees. It was earlier seen mainly in postmenopausal women. However, in 2–14% of cases, it occurs in young women (<40 years), most of whom wish to preserve their fertility.[1]

Hence, oncofertility plays a role. Usually, in these women, the cancer is an estrogen-sensitive well-differentiated endometroid carcinoma.

Over the years with early diagnosis and improved treatment, the survival rate of women with endometrial cancer has improved. Hence, their quality of life becomes important after cancer remission. A very important aspect of quality of life is to be able to have children and a family. Fertility preservation before cancer becomes an important part of oncology treatment. However, it cannot be recommended to all these patients and a criterion of selection needs to be followed.

Women at risk of endometrial cancer are those who are obese, taking estrogen therapy, tamoxifen, or those with polycystic ovarian syndrome (PCOS) or endometrial hyperplasia.

Treatment option for women with endometrial cancer desirous of pregnancy:
- Complete surgery with gamete cryopreservation and surrogacy
- *Fertility preservation:*
  - Medical (hormonal) management and assisted reproductive technology (ART)
    - Counseling
    - Informed consent
    - Concerns during controlled ovarian stimulation (COS)
    - ART outcome
  - Medical (hormonal) management and natural pregnancy.

■ SELECTION OF PATIENTS FOR FERTILITY PRESERVATION

There are certain prerequisites laid down by the oncologist which should be fulfilled in order to advise conservative treatment needed for fertility preservation. The patient must be evaluated by the fertility specialist and oncologist to ensure that the patient is appropriate for fertility treatment planned after preservation. Multidisciplinary discussions are ideal in such cases.

The essential prerequisites from the oncologist's perspective are as follows:
- Early stage cancer must be confined to the endometrium [stage 1A—International Federation of Gynecology and Obstetrics (FIGO)]. Magnetic resonance imaging (MRI), computed tomography (CT) scan, and pelvic ultrasound (transabdominal and transvaginal) are done for evaluation.[2]
- Cancer on histopathology should be endometroid and not serous or clear cell type.
- The histopathology report of endometrium on dilation and curettage (D&C) should confirm well-differentiated cancer cells with low-grade malignancy (FIGO grade I).
- There should be no pelvic and para-aortic lymph node involvement.
- There should be no concurrent ovarian involvement.
- No contraindications to medical treatments should be present.
- The patient must strongly wish to preserve fertility and be ready for the required follow-up.
- It must be ensured that the cancer is responsive to hormonal therapy which is dependent on tumor receptor status. The response would vary from 26% to 89% in patients with estrogen-sensitive tumor and only 8–17% where it is not.[3]

Fertility evaluation by fertility specialists should include the following essential points:
- The woman should have an adequate ovarian reserve. An anti-Müllerian hormone (AMH) and antral follicle count can confirm the same.
- The uterus should be normal and there should be no contraindication to bear a pregnancy such as dense intrauterine adhesions, uterine malformations, or incompetent os.
- There should be no medical problems which contraindicate a pregnancy such as grade IV heart disease, uncontrolled diabetes, or other medical conditions.
- All other relevant factors of fertility should be thoroughly investigated such as semen analysis.

COUNSELING AND INFORMED CONSENT

When taking up a woman with endometrial carcinoma for fertility preservation and conservative treatment, appropriate counseling is needed to ensure that she understands the risks and benefits and can weigh them to take an informed decision. The counseling should be on behalf of both the oncologist and the fertility specialist.

The oncologist must explain the following:
- Inherent oncologic risks of an inadequately staged cancer as the staging is done only surgically. Since in this case no radical surgery is being done, the stage cannot be ascertained.
- The offspring can be at an increased risk of inherited malignancy.
- There could be a synchronous cancer which can be missed. Ovarian-sparing surgery should only be suggested if concurrent malignancy in ovary can be ruled out. Lynch syndrome should be kept in mind when counseling these women. Sparing the ovaries while operating is a good option in case she wants to go for in vitro fertilization (IVF) with her own oocyte taking a surrogate.[4,5]
- There is a risk of recurrence with conservative treatment since the primary lesion is not removed surgically. The 5-year recurrence-free survival rates have been shown to be 51.0%.[6]
- The patient has to be explained the need for continuous surveillance. Transvaginal ultrasound (TVS) and endometrial sampling at 4-6 months will be required.
- The need for finally going in for complete surgery after completion of family must be stressed.

The fertility specialist needs to counsel regarding expected reproductive outcomes. The patient has to be explained that the chance of pregnancy is not 100%. Appropriately informed expectations regarding reproductive potential must be given. Many patients with endometrial carcinoma face difficulty conceiving secondary to obesity, PCOS, and chronic anovulation. The options of fertility treatment ranging from natural conception to intrauterine insemination (IUI), IVF, and egg/embryo preservation are explained with their success rates. Alternative treatment with donor egg, surrogacy, or adoption must also be informed to the patient for her to take an informed decision.

FERTILITY OPTIONS AFTER CONSERVATIVE TREATMENT

After cancer treatment, a patient's fertility decision will depend on her medical status and prognosis, partner status, age, whether reproduction can occur safely for woman and offspring, and reproductive options.

NATURAL PREGNANCY, INTRAUTERINE INSEMINATION, OR IN VITRO FERTILIZATION?

Successful natural pregnancy after conservative treatment can occur. She should be counseled to go for IVF as it has the highest chance of pregnancy in the shortest time, thus avoiding chances of recurrence of cancer. There is a higher pregnancy rate (PR) with ART versus natural (80.0% vs. 43.2%). The attempt to complete the family should be done in the shortest time to make the chance of recurrence minimum with definitive surgery being planned after delivery.[7] For women with partners, embryo cryopreservation is recommended. For those without partners, oocyte freezing can be done.

Controlled Ovarian Stimulation in Cases of Oncofertility

Recent studies have shown waves of folliculogenesis occur throughout the cycle. Hence, one does not wait for occurrence of menstruation to start a cycle. Random start protocols can be done at any stage of the cycle. There is an increase in estradiol levels during stimulation. It has been proposed that this may be detrimental to estrogen-sensitive tumors. Concurrent administration of aromatase inhibitors is advisable to keep estrogen levels low during stimulation. Some studies have not shown this, but it is recommended that estradiol levels are controlled with concurrent administration of aromatase inhibitors and tamoxifen. The preferred ovulation trigger is gonadotropin-releasing hormone (GnRH) agonist to prevent risk of ovarian hyperstimulation syndrome (OHSS) and high estradiol.[8]

For those undergoing complete surgery, oocyte cryopreservation and ovarian tissue cryopreservation are viable options. *Ovarian tissue cryopreservation* is still experimental and requires ovarian tissue transplantation at a later date. Some pregnancies have been reported.[9-11]

The American Society of Assisted Reproduction (ASRM) recognizes oocyte freezing as a procedure with equally good results.[12]

■ ETHICAL AND LEGAL ISSUES

There are many ethical and legal issues which need to be taken care of while preserving fertility in an endometrial cancer patient. Since these patients may have a shorter life, there should be clear directions for disposition of stored gamete and embryos in case of death. In case of posthumous reproduction, consent is a must and should be given along with consent of the surviving spouse.

There are certain ethical questions which come up with respect to offspring. It may be considered unethical to enable persons to reproduce in situations in which the parent faces a greatly lowered lifespan or the parent's ability to care for a child is compromised. The question of a higher risk for congenital anomalies, chromosomal defects, or cancer because of previous treatment in offsprings is often asked by the patient. Preimplantation genetic testing can be recommended in case of inheritable cancers.

Period of Storage of Oocytes/Embryos

Although it is known that gametes stored for more than 30 years yielded normal pregnancy, the ART law in India states a period of 10 years as acceptable for storage of gametes and embryos. For oncofertility, rules have been relaxed for this time period with permission from the ART board.

Counseling and Support

It is important to understand the patient's dilemma. Psychological counseling becomes a must for a good oncofertility program. A counselor can settle her doubts and concerns and aid in decision-making for the patient in this difficult time.

CONSERVATIVE MEDICAL TREATMENT IN ENDOMETRIAL CANCER

These patients are put on progesterone treatment for remission of estrogen-sensitive endometrial cancers. The progesterone could be given orally in high doses or as an intrauterine device.
- Levonorgestrel intrauterine device (LNG-IUD)
- Continuous oral progesterone:
    - Oral megestrol acetate in a dose of 80–160 mg/day
    - Oral medroxy progesterone acetate (MPA) in a dose of 400–600 mg daily.

Response and Recurrence

Eighty-two percent complete and 18% partial response rates were found using the MPA regimen in a multicenter trial with only six recurrences found within 25- to 73-month follow-up.[13]

The probability of recurrence was 17.2% at 12 months and 29.2% at 24 months. LNG-IUD provides local progestin to the endometrium and spares most of the systemic effects of oral progestin, such as weight gain and increased risk of venous thrombosis.[14]

How Soon does the Therapy Show Effect?

Progestin therapy has an impact on the endometrial cells as early as 10 weeks after initiation of treatment. Most recognize the need for a minimum of 3 months of progestin therapy before assessing for a response.[15]

In a study, 73% of patients responded in 4 months to MPA. The relapse rate was found to be 36% in 22 months.[16] 28 studies containing 1,038 women were included for review and meta-analysis. Clinical remission occurred in 71% with progestins, 76% with IUD, and 87% when both were combined. With IUD alone, the recurrence rate was 9%. The best remission rates were when both routes were used in combination.

Pregnancy Outcomes

Women who took progestins alone had a PR of 34% and a live birth rate (LBR) of 20%, IUD alone showed an 18% PR and 14% LBR, and both combined showed the best results with PR of 40% and LBR of 35%. Pregnancy outcomes were lowest with IUD alone;[17,18] 50% of pregnancies were conceived by assisted reproduction.[14]

Additional Drugs Given with Progesterone

- *Metformin:* It has an effect of preventing cancer recurrence and increasing tumor radiosensitivity.
- *Tamoxifen:* It is an antiestrogen drug. Alternating progesterone and tamoxifen is an option that seems to work well and better tolerated than progesterone alone. It acts like a weak estrogen in other parts of the body preventing bone loss.
- *GnRH agonists:* These induce hypoestrogenism and may also slow the growth of cancer. Goserelin or leuprolide depot can be given every 1–3 months.
- Aromatase inhibitors.

PREGNANCY AFTER FERTILITY PRESERVATION IN ENDOMETRIAL CANCER

In vitro fertilization treatment does not increase the rate of recurrence of endometrial cancers.[19] In a review by Chao et al., 65 deliveries with 77 live births were reported. One mother died of disease after delivery. No neonatal morbidity was reported.[20]

It is important to identify the right patients for oncofertility. It is imperative to have a well-defined criterion for selection of patients with conservative treatment, a proper evaluation, and follow-up of cancer. The choice of optimum fertility treatment options must be informed to the patient.

CONCLUSION

The diagnosis of cancer is a life crisis for any patient. In a survey, most of the patients had shown a strong desire to be informed about their fertility future. They are willing to accept changes in standard protocols to preserve fertility. However, it is difficult for them to balance finances and emotions to think beyond their cancer treatment. Psychological support and counseling become an integral part of oncofertility programs for endometrial cancer patients.

KEY LEARNING POINTS

- Endometrial cancer can be conservatively managed in early stages to preserve fertility but cases need to be chosen with care.
- Oncofertility is an important part of management of young patients with endometrial cancers as survival has increased and having children directly influences quality of life.
- Counseling is essential as the patient must understand the risks of unstaged cancers, recurrence rates, need for monitoring, success and failure rates of fertility treatment, and need for surgery after completion of family.
- A multidisciplinary approach is the key to proper management in such cases.
- Legal issues such as posthumous use of gametes or rights on gametes or embryos after the death of patient must be clarified and special consents should be taken for the same.

REFERENCES

1. Fadhlaoui A, Hassouna JB, Khrouf M, Zhioua F, Chaker A. Endometrial adenocarcinoma in a 27-year-old woman. Clin Med Insights Case Rep. 2010;3:31-3.
2. Knez J, Al Mahdawi L, Takač I, Sobočan M. The perspectives of fertility preservation in women with endometrial cancer. Cancers (Basel). 2021;13(4):602.
3. Chiva L, Lapuente F, González-Cortijo L, Carballo N, García JF, Rojo A, et al. Sparing fertility in young patients with endometrial cancer. Gynecol Oncol. 2008;111:S101-4.
4. Navarria I, Usel M, Rapiti E, Neyroud-Caspar I, Pelte MF, Bouchardy C, et al. Young patients with endometrial cancer: how many could be eligible for fertility-sparing treatment? Gynecol Oncol. 2009;114:448-51.
5. Sun C, Chen G, Yang Z, Jiang J, Yang X, Li N, et al. Safety of ovarian preservation in young patients with early-stage endometrial cancer: a retrospective study and meta-analysis. Fertil Steril. 2013;100:782-7.
6. Wang CJ, Chao A, Yang LY, Hsueh S, Huang YT, Chou HH, et al. Fertility-preserving treatment in young women with endometrial adenocarcinoma: a long-term cohort study. Int J Gynecol Cancer. 2014;24(4):718-28.
7. Tong XM, Lin XN, Jiang HF, Jiang LY, Zhang SY, Liang FB. Fertility-preserving treatment and pregnancy outcomes in the early stage of endometrial carcinoma. Chin Med J (Engl). 2013;126(15):2965-71.
8. Oktay K, Türkçüoğlu I, Rodriguez-Wallberg KA. GnRH agonist trigger for women with breast cancer undergoing fertility preservation by aromatase inhibitor/FSH stimulation. Reprod Biomed Online. 2010;20:783-8.
9. Lotz L, Maktabi A, Hoffmann I, Findeklee S, Beckmann MW, Dittrich R. Ovarian tissue cryopreservation and retransplantation—what do patients think about it? Reprod Biomed Online. 2016;32(4):394-400.
10. Salama M, Woodruff TK. New advances in ovarian autotransplantation to restore fertility in cancer patients. Cancer Metastasis Rev. 2015;34:807-22.
11. Practice Committee of American Society for Reproductive Medicine. Ovarian tissue cryopreservation: a committee opinion. Fertil Steril. 2014;101:1237-43.
12. Cobo A, Meseguer M, Remohí J, Pellicer A. Use of cryo-banked oocytes in an ovum donation programme: a prospective, randomized, controlled, clinical trial. Hum. Reprod. 2010;25(9):2239-46.
13. Kim JJ, Chapman-Davis E. Role of progesterone in endometrial cancer. Semin Reprod Med. 2010;28(1):81-90.
14. Kozaks M, Uman J, Luton D, Rouser R, Darian E. Prognostic factors of oncologic and reproductive outcomes in fertility-sparing management of endometrial atypical hyperplasia and adenocarcinoma: systematic review and meta-analysis. Fertil Steril. 2014;101:785-94.
15. Pronin SM, Novikova OV, Andreeva JY, Novikova EG. Fertility-sparing treatment of early endometrial cancer and complex atypical hyperplasia in young women of childbearing potential. Int J Gynecol Cancer. 2015;25:1010-4.
16. Kalogiannidis I, Agorastos T. Conservative management of young patients with endometrial highly-differentiated adenocarcinoma. J Obstet Gynaecol. 2011;31:13-7.

17. Wei J, Zhang W, Feng L, Gao W. Comparison of fertility-sparing treatments in patients with early endometrial cancer and atypical complex hyperplasia: a meta-analysis and systematic review. Medicine (Baltimore). 2017;96(37):e8034.
18. Guillon S, Popescu N, Phelippeau J, Koskas M. A systematic review and meta-analysis of prognostic factors for remission in fertility-sparing management of endometrial atypical hyperplasia and adenocarcinoma. Int J Gynaecol Obstet. 2019;146(3):277-88.
19. Vougon M, Peigné M, Phelippeau J, Gonthier C, Koskas M, et al. IVF impact on the risk of recurrence of endometrial adenocarcinoma after fertility-sparing management. Reprod Biomed Online. 2021;43(3):495-502.
20. Chao AS, Chao A, Wang CJ, Lai CH, Wang HS. Obstetric outcomes of pregnancy after conservative treatment of endometrial cancer: case series and literature review. Taiwan J Obstet Gynecol. 2011;50(1):62-6.

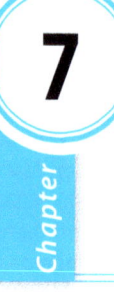

Fertility and Assisted Reproductive Technology in Cancer Survivors: Hereditary Cancers

Roya Rozati, Wajeeda Tabasum, Naila Mohiuddin

■ INTRODUCTION

Cancers can either be sporadic, which accounts for 80-90%, or hereditary, which accounts for 5-10%. Sporadic cancers result from spontaneous and induced mutations,[1] while hereditary cancers are caused by germline mutations.[2]

It is a genetic predisposition to certain cancer forms that usually manifests in childhood due to inherited pathogenic mutations in one or more genes. Concerns about the children accompany parenting in affected women, which is typical of the autosomal dominant inheritance.

An estimated 5-10% of all cancer diagnoses are caused by hereditary cancer genetic predisposition syndromes resulting from inherited pathogenic mutations in one or more genes.[3,4]

Hereditary cancer is usually associated with germline mutations and it can be transmitted to offspring through maternal or paternal lineage.[5]

Breast, ovarian, endometrial, and colon cancer are frequently seen by obstetrician-gynecologist care providers and may be a component of a particular hereditary cancer syndrome. The onset of cancer often occurs at an early age, and families frequently exhibit an inheritance pattern.[6]

It may be helpful to identify families at risk for particular cancers early in order to determine whether those screenings and risk-reducing measures should be conducted earlier[7-9] and more thoroughly. When a patient has breast or ovarian cancer, reproductive choices, fertility decisions, and family building decisions are significantly impacted.[9]

The majority of women with inherited cancers include breast and ovarian cancers which carry a deleterious mutation of *BRCA1*, *BRAC2*, *CDH1*, *PALB2*, *PTEN*, and *TP53*, among others that are associated with hereditary risk.[10]

A genetic pathogenic gene variation increases the risk of gynecologic cancer in women, so it is important to discuss the risks of passing hereditary pathogenic gene variants on to future generations as well as the possibility of hormone therapy after oophorectomy that reduces risk.[9]

Cancer survival rates have resulted in more women not having children at the time of cancer diagnosis and having an option of fertility preservation.[11] An oncofertility combined with oncology and reproductive treatment options expands fertility preservation options in cancer survivors.[12,13]

FAMILY AND MEDICAL HISTORY SCREENING

Hereditary cancer often occurs earlier than a sporadic form of cancer, so screening at a younger age is recommended. The cornerstone to identifying patients and families that have a higher chance of contracting a particular type of cancer is a hereditary cancer risk assessment. At the time of diagnosis, a family history should be obtained and updated as needed. Pedigree analysis is a key component to consider. First-degree relatives are siblings, parents, and children. The second degree of relation includes grandparents, aunts, uncles, grandchildren, nieces, nephews, and half-siblings. With each case of cancer in the family, the maternal and paternal sides of Ashkenazi heritage determine the age of cancer diagnosis and the primary cancer type.

A possible hereditary cancer syndrome can be identified by specific characteristics reflecting personal or family medical history.
- When a patient is abnormally young or under 50 years old, a diagnosis of breast, ovarian, or colon cancer is made.
- Many close relatives from the same family side suffer from the same type of cancer (e.g., a mother, daughter, and sister all have breast cancer).
- A single patient has a variety of cancers.
- Several primary tumors in one individual, frequently in the same organ (such as the colon or breast).
- An unusual presentation of a particular cancer type (e.g., a male with breast cancer).
- Certain benign conditions, such as skin growths or skeletal abnormalities, are associated with inherited cancer syndromes.

The probability of hereditary cancer syndrome is high when:
- There is a 30% incidence of triple-negative breast cancer among women who are <60 years old. These patients lack the expression of estrogen and progesterone receptors and there is no overexpression of ERBB2 (also known as HER2 or HER2/neu). This may suggest a hereditary breast and ovarian cancer syndrome.[14]
- The histology of ovarian, fallopian tube, or peritoneal cancers is predominantly serous (suggesting hereditary breast and ovarian cancer syndrome, which affects 10–15% of women).[15]
- Colorectal cancer that has a deoxyribonucleic acid (DNA) mismatch repair defect [suggesting Lynch syndrome (24%)].[16]
- Endometrial cancer with a defective DNA mismatch repair system (suggesting Lynch syndrome (12%)].[17]

Preconception Counseling

Preconception counseling includes fertility issues, the role of preimplantation genetic testing, and genetic counseling.

As part of preconception counseling, family medical history, including those of family members who have never developed cancer, is reviewed to ensure patient comprehension and ease in delivering results.

Counseling women on the age-specific, primary site, and cumulative risks of hereditary cancers and preventive strategies can assist in decision-making. Fertility preservation to prevent cancer treatments' detrimental effects differs from other clinical contexts. The necessity to preserve gametes is indeed predictable and expected to be common. We support individualized and early fertility counseling for these reasons. Carriers need to understand the possibility of transmission. It is important to explore whether elective oocyte cryopreservation can be done before (for previvors) or after (for survivors) cancer diagnosis. The alternatives for preimplantation genetic testing (PGT) and oocyte donation should also be explained to them.

One of the research studies concluded that out of 150 live births, one newborn is affected with chromosomal abnormalities, and approximately 5–7% of children die due to chromosomal defects.[18] PGT, which includes preimplantation genetic diagnosis (PGD), can precisely detect chromosomal abnormalities.[19] Most of the participants consider PGT as their only possible reproductive choice. PGT helps us to minimize or reduce the risk of transmission of the genetic mutation to the fetus. In in vitro fertilization (IVF), this procedure allows the transfer of unaffected embryos that have been genetically tested after IVF. Providing comprehensive care to young women with hereditary breast and ovarian cancer requires raising awareness about PGD and its benefits. A fetus will be examined for the presence of a genetic mutation during prenatal diagnosis. Regardless of the couple's fertility, IVF/intracytoplasmic sperm injection (ICSI) treatment is required for PGT. Moreover, the chance of conception with IVF/ICSI is limited even among normally fertile couples, given the pregnancy rate.[20] Prior to engaging in pretext genetic counseling, patients are advised to speak with a licensed genetic counselor or another genetics expert. The family history is widened through genetic counseling, and the possibility to uncover impacts other than common cancers, effects on family members, and incidental findings with ambiguous clinical importance is examined.

For couples with hereditary cancers, making reproductive decisions about PGT has proven to be an extremely difficult and stressful process. We found that the couples' perceptions of the significance of the tendency and their moral perspectives on selection served as the key guiding principles. For female carriers, it was crucial that IVF be safe and that the PGT planning procedure work with preventive surgeries. Hence, clinical geneticists and couples at risk for hereditary cancer are involved in oncogenetic counseling regarding the development, which will aid the patient in making an appropriate patient decision for reproductive choices.

PATHOGENIC VARIANTS IN HEREDITARY CANCER GENES AND FERTILITY PRESERVATION

Young women with hereditary cancer who carry germline pathogenic variants are similarly concerned about future fertility and are likely to pursue fertility preservation as noncarriers. Concern about cancer risk heritability was common among carriers and noncarriers desiring future fertility, suggesting a gap between perceived and actual risk. All women diagnosed at reproductive age should be counseled about genetic counseling, which ought to be an integral component of fertility preservation.[21,22]

Concerns during ART—Due to High Estradiol Levels in Controlled Ovarian Stimulation, any Special Precautions during ART

Recent assisted reproductive technology (ART) treatments behold mild ovarian stimulation regimens, which are more individualized depending on ovarian reserve.[23] Many women who are more likely to get these cancers are concerned about how ovarian stimulation's high estradiol levels would affect their cancer susceptibility. The risk of mutation carriers does not appear to be increased by fertility medications.[24] Most ovarian hyperstimulation syndrome (OHSS) is mild and of little clinical concern. Severe OHSS can lead to significant morbidity and mortality.[25] OHSS is a complication associated with controlled ovarian stimulation (COS) which clinicians have no complete way of preventing at present. It begins with the identification of the "high-risk" woman through to the woman who is "at risk" and subsequently initiating the appropriate therapies such as reducing gonadotropin dose, duration, gonadotropin-releasing hormone agonist (GnRHa) as an ovulation trigger, adjuvant metformin therapy, cabergoline, and cryopreservation—utilized as clinically appropriate.

Assisted Reproductive Technology: Any Special Concerns in Women with Hereditary Cancers

Concerns about breast, ovarian, or uterine cancer risk are associated with artificial reproduction technology. The primary aim for performing PGT was to prevent their genetic disorder in future offspring. To decide to undergo PGT was perceived by the couples as the means to take control over their child's genetic status and their reproductive reality. There is no evidence to suggest that fertility drugs are associated with an increased risk of breast or ovarian cancer at present.[26] Individuals who do not want this mutation to be transferred to their offspring need to go screening through PGD through IVF/ICSI, where embryos for the genetic mutation will be screened, and only unaffected embryos will be transferred. Parenthood in women carrying hereditary cancer syndrome is a multifaceted and intricate issue.

■ OBSTETRIC OUTCOME—TRANSMISSION CHANCES

Genetic counseling and testing can be provided to patients with familial cancer syndromes by obstetrician-gynecologist in addition to potentially life-saving measures to reduce cancer risk. For women at risk for hereditary gynecologic malignancies, chemotherapy and risk-reducing surgery can reduce cancer risk, but these measures may also affect fertility and hormone function. It is likely that additional management options will be available for at-risk people and couples as genetic testing becomes more accessible and ART advances.

MANAGEMENT STRATEGIES FOR HEREDITARY CANCER SYNDROME

- Proper genetic counseling should be given
- Reproductive options should be given such as PGD, aneuploidy testing, and third-party reproduction, and screening of individuals should be done.
- The following intervention should be followed: Lifestyle modification, pharmacological treatment (chemoprevention), and surgical management.

■ CONCLUSION

With chemotherapy and risk-reducing surgeries, hereditary gynecological cancers can be prevented, but these treatments may affect hormones and reproductive function in the future. Women can use a variety of family building and fertility preservation techniques to meet their reproductive goals, including adoption, gestational carriers, donor oocytes, donor embryos, and cryopreservation of embryos and/or oocytes.

Before embryo transfer or during pregnancy, genetic testing can be used to find out if embryos or newborns have a gene mutation. This reduces the likelihood of transmission.

KEY LEARNING POINTS

- Hereditary gynecological cancers raise concerns about cancer prevention, early detection, fertility, and hormonal health. Few options are used to lower the risk of gynecologic cancer, but many of them can cause infertility and surgically accelerated menopause.
- Fertility preservation and family building techniques including gestational carriers, donor oocytes, donor embryos, and oocyte and embryo cryopreservation can be used to assist women to achieve their reproductive goals.
- Genetic testing can be performed prior to embryo transfer or during pregnancy to determine if an embryo or fetus suffers from a detrimental gene mutation. Through genetic testing, the risk of transmission can be reduced.
- It is possible to consider hormone therapy as a precautionary measure for surgically menopausal women without a personal history of breast cancer.

■ REFERENCES

1. Lu Y, Ek WE, Whiteman D, Vaughan TL, Spurdle AB, Easton DF, et al. Most common 'sporadic' cancers have a significant germline genetic component. Hum Mol Genet. 2014;23(22):6112-8.
2. Ngeow J, Eng C. Precision medicine in heritable cancer: when somatic tumour testing and germline mutations meet. NPJ Genom Med. 2016;1(1):15006.
3. Nagy R, Sweet K, Eng C. Highly penetrant hereditary cancer syndromes. Oncogene. 2004;23(38):6445-70.
4. Garber JE, Offit K. Hereditary cancer predisposition syndromes. J Clin Oncol. 2005;23(2):276-92.
5. Antoniou A, Pharoah PD, Narod S, Risch HA, Eyfjord JE, Hopper JL, et al. Average risks of breast and ovarian cancer associated with BRCA1 or BRCA2 mutations detected in case series unselected for family history: a combined analysis of 22 studies. Am J Hum Genet. 2003;72(5):1117-30.
6. Lynch HT, Watson P, Conway TA, Lynch JF. Clinical/genetic features in hereditary breast cancer. Breast Cancer Res Treat. 1990;15:63-71.
7. Loud JT, Murphy J. Cancer screening and early detection in the 21st century. Semin Oncol Nurs. 2017;33(2):121-8.
8. Rubinstein WS, Acheson LS, O'Neill SM, Ruffin 4th MT, Wang C, Beaumont JL, et al. Clinical utility of family history for cancer screening and referral in primary care: a report from the Family Healthware Impact Trial. Genet Med. 2011;13(11):956-65.
9. Chen LM, Blank SV, Burton E, Glass K, Penick E, Woodard T. Reproductive and hormonal considerations in women at increased risk for hereditary gynecologic cancers: Society of Gynecologic Oncology and American Society for Reproductive Medicine evidence-based review. Gynecol Oncol. 2019;155(3):508-14.
10. Peshkin BN, Isaacs CC, Goff B, Burstein HJ. Overview of hereditary breast and ovarian cancer syndromes associated with genes other than BRCA1/2. Waltham, MA: UpToDate; 2021.
11. Jeruss JS, Woodruff TK. Preservation of fertility in patients with cancer. N Engl J Med. 2009;360(9):902-11.
12. Woodruff TK. Oncofertility: a grand collaboration between reproductive medicine and oncology. Reproduction. 2015;150(3):S1-10.
13. Rashedi AS, de Roo SF, Ataman LM, Edmonds ME, Silva AA, Scarella A, et al. Survey of fertility preservation options available to patients with cancer around the globe. JCO Glob Oncol. 2020;6:331-44.
14. Greenup R, Buchanan A, Lorizio W, Rhoads K, Chan S, Leedom T, et al. Prevalence of BRCA mutations among women with triple-negative breast cancer (TNBC) in a genetic counseling cohort. Ann Surg Oncol. 2013;20:3254-8.
15. Risch HA, McLaughlin JR, Cole DE, Rosen B, Bradley L, Kwan E, et al. Prevalence and penetrance of germline BRCA1 and BRCA2 mutations in a population series of 649 women with ovarian cancer. Am J Hum Genet. 2001;68(3):700-10.
16. Moreira L, Balaguer F, Lindor N, de la Chapelle A, Hampel H, Aaltonen LA, et al. Identification of Lynch syndrome among patients with colorectal cancer. JAMA. 2012;308(15):1555-65.
17. Dillon JL, Gonzalez JL, DeMars L, Bloch KJ, Tafe LJ. Universal screening for Lynch syndrome in endometrial cancers: frequency of germline mutations and identification of patients with Lynch-like syndrome. Hum Pathol. 2017;70:121-8.

18. Nussbaum RL, McInnes RR, Willard HF (Eds). Thompson & Thompson Genetics in Medicine. Philadelphia, PA: WB Saunders; 2001. 464 pp.
19. Simpson JL, Kuliev A, Rechitsky S. Overview of preimplantation genetic diagnosis (PGD): historical perspective and future direction. Methods Mol Biol. 2019;1885:23-43.
20. Ferraretti AP, Goossens V, de Mouzon J, Bhattacharya S, Castilla JA, Korsak V, et al. Assisted reproductive technology in Europe, 2008: results generated from European registers by ESHRE. Hum Reprod. 2012;27(9):2571-84.
21. Lewinsohn RM, Zheng Y, Rosenberg SM, Ruddy KJ, Tamimi R, Schapira L, et al. Fertility preferences, concerns, and preservation among young women with breast cancer who carry germline genetic pathogenic variants compared with non-carriers. J Clin Oncol. 2022;40(16 Suppl.):10607.
22. Buonomo B, Massarotti C, Dellino M, Anserini P, Ferrari A, Campanella M, et al. Reproductive issues in carriers of germline pathogenic variants in the BRCA1/2 genes: an expert meeting. BMC Med. 2021;19(1):205.
23. Tan BK, Mathur R. Management of ovarian hyperstimulation syndrome. Produced on behalf of the BFS policy and practice committee. Hum Fertil (Camb). 2013;16(3):151-9.
24. Practice Committee of the American Society for Reproductive Medicine. Fertility drugs and cancer: a guideline. Fertil Steril. 2016;106(7):1617-26.
25. Nelson SM. Prevention and management of ovarian hyperstimulation syndrome. Thromb Res. 2017;151:S61-4.
26. Gronwald J, Glass K, Rosen B, Karlan B, Tung N, Neuhausen SL, et al. Treatment of infertility does not increase the risk of ovarian cancer among women with a BRCA1 or BRCA2 mutation. Fertil Steril. 2016;105(3):781-5.

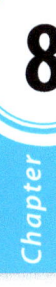

Fertility and Assisted Reproductive Technology in Cancer Survivors: Lymphoma/Leukemia

Pankaj Talwar, Shahida Naghma

■ INTRODUCTION

Oncofertility is the wider advanced branch of reproductive medicine which provides fertility preservation options for young cancer patients. Infertility is a growing health concern worldwide. With the advent of newer and efficient diagnostic tools, the timely diagnosis and treatment of various cancers have increased the longevity of young cancer survivors. But the impact of cancer treatment on fertility can be long-lasting. It can even lead to fertility loss in severe cases.[1,2] In women, hematological malignancies account for 7–9% of estimated new cancer cases and deaths. The most common forms occurring in girls and young women are acute lymphocytic leukemia (ALL), acute myeloid leukemia (AML), non-Hodgkin's lymphoma (NHL), and Hodgkin's lymphoma (HL) and hence necessitates fertility preservation.

■ RISK OF GONADOTOXICITY

The alkylating drugs used in chemotherapy and total body irradiation (TBI) are associated with the risks of gonadotoxicity and can lead to iatrogenic premature ovarian insufficiency (POI) and fertility loss. This risk is dependent on the type and dose of therapy given and the type and stage of cancer.

The latest European Society of Human Reproduction and Embryology (ESHRE) guidelines recommend assessing the risk of gonadotoxicity in all patients undergoing gonadotoxic treatments[3] and hence the need for and emphasis on counseling and explaining the currently available fertility preservation options for patients.[4-6]

■ FERTILITY PRESERVATION OPTIONS FOR FEMALE PATIENTS WITH HEMATOLOGICAL MALIGNANCIES

The overall 5-year survival rates in hematological malignancies have increased, quoted around 60% for leukemia and 80% for lymphoma.[7] The fertility preservation options as outlined by the latest ESHRE guidelines are divided into established, debatable, and experimental (**Flowchart 1**).[1] Embryo freezing and oocyte freezing are the established methods of fertility preservation being widely utilized. Debatable options may include ovarian protection techniques such as gonadotropin-releasing hormone

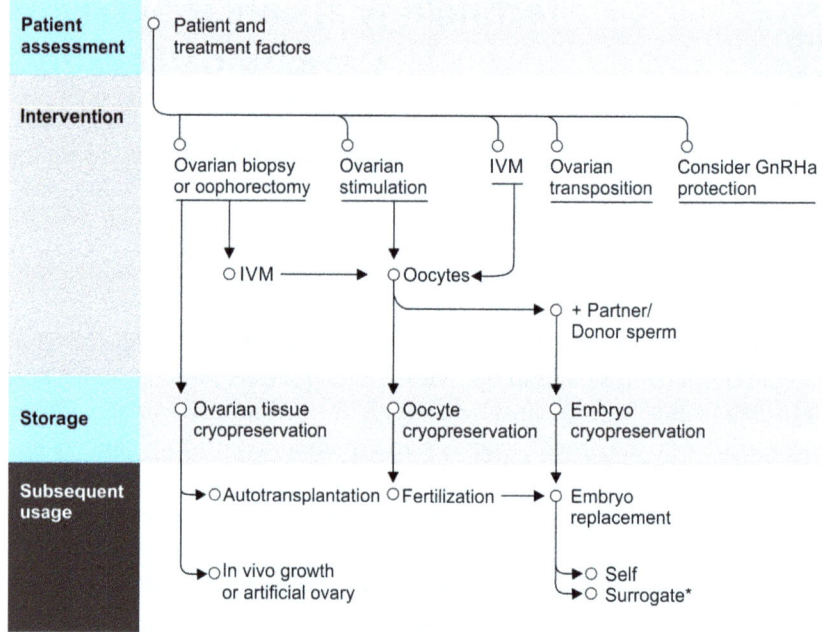

Flowchart 1: Fertility preservation options in female patients.

(GnRHa: gonadotropin-releasing hormone agonist; IVM: in vitro maturation)
*Surrogate: pertaining to local guidelines on surrogacy
Source: Anderson et al. (2015).[1]

(GnRH) analogs and hormonal suppression, surgical ovarian transposition (oophoropexy), and gonadal shielding. Methods such as ovarian tissue freezing and further autotransplantation, oocyte in vitro maturation (IVM), artificial ovary, stem cells, and neoadjuvant cytoprotective pharmacotherapy are still in an experimental phase.[8-11] The best-suited guidelines for fertility preservation have been given lately by ESHRE in the year 2020,[3] while the others being American Society of Clinical Oncology (ASCO),[12-14] American Society for Reproductive Medicine (ASRM),[15,16] European Society for Medical Oncology (ESMO),[17,18] American Oncofertility Consortium (OC),[19,20] International Society for Fertility Preservation (ISFP),[21-24] National Comprehensive Cancer Network (NCCN),[25] and American Academy of Pediatrics (AAP) for childhood malignancies.[26]

Established Options

Embryo Freezing

For years now, embryo freezing has been the gold-standard option for female fertility preservation. This method is well suited in patients because of its ease, safety, short time, and feasibility in urgent situations.[3] It involves cryopreservation of in vitro-fertilized mature oocytes via vitrification.[27]

Embryo freezing involves gonadotropin injections for ovarian stimulation, oocyte retrieval, and sperm for in vitro fertilization (IVF). Therefore, it is not suited for prepubertal girls and single women. It is also not suitable in the case of estrogen-sensitive cancers, such as breast and endometrial cancers, as conventional ovarian stimulation may lead to high serum estrogen levels. In such cases, which are at high risk of estrogen exposure, ovarian stimulation can be done with either tamoxifen (selective estrogen receptor modulator)[28,29] or letrozole (aromatase inhibitor).[30,31] Highly aggressive malignancies that require immediate anticancer treatment such as leukemia can benefit more from random-start ovarian stimulation protocol for emergency fertility preservation.[32-34] Most of the laboratory centers store frozen embryos, eggs, and sperm for 10 years, although longer storage periods may be possible depending on differences in local and national regulations in different countries. In female patients with cancer, the live birth rate per frozen embryo transfer may be reduced due to additional harmful effects of radiotherapy/chemotherapy.[35]

Egg Freezing

Egg or oocyte freezing is no longer an experimental method for female fertility preservation.[3,36] It involves cryopreservation of mature oocytes via vitrification.[37-39] Egg freezing involves gonadotropin-induced ovarian stimulation followed by oocyte retrieval without the need for sperm or IVF. It remains unsuitable for prepubertal girls due to immature hypothalamic-pituitary ovarian axis but can be used for single women. The precautions and disadvantages of this procedure are the same as embryo freezing as both involve controlled ovarian hyperstimulation to obtain the oocytes.

Debatable Options

Gonadotropin-releasing Hormone Analogs and Hormonal Suppression

There is still debate around the protective use of GnRH analogs before and during chemotherapy. Although few studies have shown a correlation between the use of GnRH analogs and lower rates of POI in young female cancer patients, large multicentric trials are needed to establish and understand this further.[40-44] GnRH analogs suppress gonadotropin secretion from the pituitary gland by feedback mechanism which suppresses ovarian function indirectly. The ovaries in this suppressed state decrease the primordial follicles entering the growing pool, making them less sensitive to gonadotoxic chemotherapy. Other mechanisms include upregulation of intraovarian antiapoptotic molecules and protection of ovarian germline stem cells. GnRH analogs do not protect ovaries from radiotherapy-induced gonadotoxicity; hence, it is not feasible to use in patients scheduled to receive pelvic, abdominal, or TBI. Hence, GnRH analog use is still debatable.[45]

Oophoropexy

In cases of malignancies with pelvic involvement, the ovaries are moved away from the field of pelvic irradiation such as in HL, cervical carcinoma, vaginal carcinoma, and pelvic sarcoma. Oophoropexy can be done via minilaparotomy, laparoscopy, or through robotic surgery. If preferred, in the same surgical setting, oophoropexy can be carried out to one ovary and ovarian tissue cryopreservation (OTC) from the other ovary.[46] Oophoropexy still remains debatable as it does not protect ovaries from chemotherapy-induced gonadotoxicity.[12-14]

Gonadal Shielding

Gonadal shielding can be used during pelvic irradiation to provide some ovarian protection, especially in young patients. Since it does not protect ovaries from chemotherapy-induced gonadotoxicity, it has limited role when chemotherapy is given.[12-14]

Another important limitation in using oophoropexy and gonadal shielding is in case of hematologic malignancies which have spread to ovaries through bloodstream.

Experimental Options

Ovarian Tissue Cryopreservation and Autotransplantation

Ovarian tissue freezing involves cryopreservation of surgically extracted cortical ovarian tissues.[47-50] Before starting the anticancer treatment, at least half of one ovary is excised via laparoscopy or laparotomy. This ovarian tissue can be transported within 24 hours to central cryobanks to be processed by experienced oncofertility teams. Immature oocytes can be retrieved from this extracted ovarian tissue for IVM and vitrification. The slow-freezing protocol is well established and considered as standard for OTC.[3] Before proceeding with ovarian tissue transplantation, the ovarian tissue should be evaluated for the presence of residual malignant cells in the ovarian cortex (and in the residual medulla when available). The same should be said prior to OTC, all risks explained.[3] Thawed ovarian tissue can be transplanted back either to the remaining ovary or ovarian fossa (orthotopic transplantation) or to any other site such as subcutaneous space of the abdominal wall or forearm (heterotopic transplantation). Ovaries can become functional 2-9 months postoperatively and may last years after. Since no prior ovarian stimulation is needed, the cancer treatment does not get delayed. Moreover, this option can also restore both endocrine and reproductive ovarian functions following cancer treatment. To avoid reintroducing malignant cells, ovarian tissue transplantation (OTT) should be absolutely contraindicated in all types of ovarian cancers and high-risk leukemia.[51,52] Although this new result is very remarkable, it is inconclusive for all leukemia patients and seems to be case-dependent and should therefore be extrapolated with extreme caution.

In Vitro Maturation of Oocytes

It is an innovative fertility preservation (FP) procedure.[3] Immature oocytes can also be retrieved from unstimulated ovaries through an ultrasound-guided transvaginal approach. These oocytes should be cultured further in vitro for 24–48 hours for them to mature into metaphase II (MII) oocytes and can be used readily for IVF or vitrification.[53,54] It is feasible for prepubertal girls as well.

Artificial Ovary

Artificial ovary is a novel experimental technology that aims to produce mature oocytes ready for IVF through an ex vivo multistep strategy including sequential in vitro cultures of ovarian tissue, follicles, and oocytes.[55-58] Although currently under an experimental phase, further advances in research will improve the results and make it possible for transposition to human models.

Stem Cells Reproductive Technologies

The recent advances in stem cells research and discovery of ovarian (oogonial) stem cells (OSCs) and induced pluripotent stem cells (iPSCs) have paved the way for more fertility options for cancer survivors.[59-61]

WHAT ARE THE ASSISTED REPRODUCTIVE TECHNOLOGY OPTIONS POST-TREATMENT OF HEMATOLOGICAL CANCERS?

Elevated serum estradiol (E_2) levels pose a major issue during stimulations in estrogen-sensitive cancers as it may promote growth of tumors, such as endometrial and estrogen-receptor-positive breast cancers.[62] But for most hematological malignancies, this concern does not arise. Hence, conventional controlled ovarian stimulation (COS) protocols can be used depending on the patient's ovarian reserve post cancer therapy. The final success rate depends upon the quantity and quality of the patient's present ovarian reserve.

Prior to embryo transfer, a thorough assessment of fitness for pregnancy is recommended to predict and prevent possible complications.[3] There is always a need for psychological, preconception, and fertility treatment counseling for all patients.

Comprehensive Multidisciplinary Fertility Preservation and Restoration Strategy for Girls and Young Women with Hematological Malignancies

There is an increased risk of developing obstetric and birth complications in terms of an increased risk of prematurity [relative risk (RR) 1.56; 95% confidence interval (CI) 1.37–1.77], low birth weight (RR 1.47; 95% CI 1.24–1.73), elective (RR 1.38; 95% CI 1.13–1.70) and emergency cesarean section (RR 1.22; 95% CI 1.15–1.30), assisted vaginal delivery (RR 1.10; 95% CI 1.02–1.18), and postpartum hemorrhage (RR 1.18; 95% CI 1.02–1.36).[63]

The risk of these complications appears to be higher when the interval between the end of treatment and conception is short.[64] Therefore, close monitoring of post-treatment pregnancies and an interval of at least 1 year following completion of chemotherapy is recommended in cancer survivors. In patients receiving other anticancer treatments, a specific washout period should be considered before conception.

FERTILITY PRESERVATION OPTIONS IN MALE PATIENTS WITH HEMATOLOGICAL MALIGNANCIES

The severity of the testicular damage occurring during cancer treatment varies and mostly depends on the type, cumulative dose of chemotherapeutic drugs, duration, site of irradiation, and fractionation schedule of radiotherapy.[65-67] Another important factor remains the patient's age and susceptibility of organs to treatment.[68]

The first-line standard method in male fertility preservation is collection and cryopreservation of mature spermatozoa. Multiple semen samples should be cryopreserved. This method is not applicable when the patient cannot produce a sperm sample, for example, azoospermic males prior to cancer treatment or prepubertal males.

For pubertal males who cannot provide a sperm sample by masturbation, assistance can be provided in the form of penile vibratory stimulation or electroejaculation under general anesthesia to retrieve sperm and freeze. Sperm can also be obtained via testicular sperm extraction (TESE) in cases of azoospermia.[69] If none of the above techniques are successful, or not possible like in the case of prepubertal males, testicular tissue (TT) can be excised and banked to preserve the spermatogonial stem cells (SSCs).[70]

Following TT cryopreservation, the three fertility restoration methods currently being studied under development are (1) autotransplantation of the TT, (2) autotransplantation of isolated SSCs from TT, and (3) in vitro spermatogenesis.[71,72] Keeping the risk of reintroducing tumor cells in mind, TT is not recommended for patients who suffered from childhood hematological cancers or metastatic malignancies. For these patients, SSC propagation and autotransplantation of SSCs appear to be a better option as the malignant cells could be eliminated during the cell sorting process.[68]

CONCLUSION

One in six couples worldwide, accounting for 17.5% of adult population, experiences infertility.[73] There is hence an urgent need to provide better fertility preservation options to patients tailored according to their needs. Patients facing cancer should be informed about their reproductive risks and options to reduce distress and improve their quality of life.

A comprehensive multidisciplinary fertility team should be designed to address the needs of patients diagnosed with carcinoma.

KEY LEARNING POINTS
- With recent advances in medical field, the longevity of young cancer survivors has increased.
- Better fertility preservation technique is required to meet this unmet need.
- Embryo and sperm cryopreservation have been the well-established methods.
- Latest ESHRE guidelines quote oocyte freezing as an established method of fertility preservation.
- A comprehensive approach with adequate information about the risks pertaining to ovarian stimulation, oocyte retrieval and risks associated with pregnancy post cancer treatments, should be provided.

REFERENCES

1. Anderson RA, Mitchell RT, Kelsey TW, Spears N, Telfer EE, Wallace WHB. Cancer treatment and gonadal function: experimental and established strategies for fertility preservation in children and young adults. Lancet Diabetes Endocrinol. 2015;3(7):556-67.
2. Kort JD, Eisenberg ML, Millheiser LS, Westphal LM. Fertility issues in cancer survivorship. CA Cancer J Clin. 2014;64(2):118-34.
3. The ESHRE Guideline Group on Female Fertility Preservation, Anderson RA, Amant F, Braat D, D'Angelo A, de Sousa Lopes SMC, et al. ESHRE guideline: female fertility preservation. Hum Reprod Open. 2020;2020(4):hoaa052.
4. Shapira M, Raanani H, Cohen Y, Meirow D. Fertility preservation in young females with hematological malignancies. Acta Haematol. 2014;132(3-4):400-13.
5. Loren AW. Fertility issues in patients with hematologic malignancies. Hematology Am Soc Hematol Educ Program. 2015;2015(1):138-45.
6. Anderson RA, Remedios R, Kirkwood AA, Patrick P, Stevens L, Clifton-Hadley L, et al. Determinants of ovarian function after response-adapted therapy in patients with advanced Hodgkin's lymphoma (RATHL): a secondary analysis of a randomized phase 3 trial. Lancet Oncol. 2018;19(10):1328-37.
7. Howlader N, Noone AM, Krapcho M, Miller D, Bishop K, Altekruse SF, et al. (Eds). SEER (Surveillance, Epidemiology and End Results) Cancer Statistics Review, 1975-2013. Bethesda, MD: National Cancer Institute; 2016.

8. Salama M, Winkler K, Murach KF, Seeber B, Ziehr SC, Wildt L. Female fertility loss and preservation: threats and opportunities. Ann Oncol. 2013;24(3):598-608.
9. De Vos M, Smitz J, Woodruff TK. Fertility preservation in women with cancer. Lancet. 2014;384(9950):1302-10.
10. Metzger ML, Meacham LR, Patterson B, Casillas JS, Constine LS, Hijiya N, et al. Female reproductive health after childhood, adolescent, and young adult cancers: guidelines for the assessment and management of female reproductive complications. J Clin Oncol. 2013;31(9):1239-47.
11. Dolmans MM, Lambertini M, Macklon KT, Santos TA, Ruiz-Casado A, Borini A, et al. EUropean REcommendations for female FERtility preservation (EU-REFER): a joint collaboration between oncologists and fertility specialists. Crit Rev Oncol Hematol. 2019;138:233-40.
12. Lee SJ, Schover LR, Partridge AH, Patrizio P, Wallace WH, Hagerty K, et al. American Society of Clinical Oncology recommendations on fertility preservation in cancer patients. J Clin Oncol. 2006;24(18):2917-31.
13. Loren AW, Mangu PB, Beck LN, Brennan L, Magdalinski AJ, Partridge AH, et al. Fertility preservation for patients with cancer: American Society of Clinical Oncology clinical practice guideline update. J Clin Oncol. 2013;31(19):2500-10.
14. Oktay K, Harvey BE, Partridge AH, Quinn GP, Reinecke J, Taylor HS, et al. Fertility preservation in patients with cancer: ASCO clinical practice guideline update. J Clin Oncol. 2018;36(19):1994-2001.
15. Ethics Committee of American Society for Reproductive Medicine. Fertility preservation and reproduction in patients facing gonadotoxic therapies: a committee opinion. Fertil Steril. 2013;100(5):1224-31.
16. Practice Committee of American Society for Reproductive Medicine. Fertility preservation in patients undergoing gonadotoxic therapy or gonadectomy: a committee opinion. Fertil Steril. 2013;100(5):1214-23.
17. Pentheroudakis G, Orecchia R, Hoekstra HJ, Pavlidis N. Cancer, fertility and pregnancy: ESMO clinical practice guidelines for diagnosis, treatment and follow-up. Ann Oncol. 2010;21(Suppl. 5):v266-73.
18. Peccatori FA, Azim Jr HA, Orecchia R, Hoekstra HJ, Pavlidis N, Kesic V, et al. Cancer, pregnancy and fertility: ESMO Clinical Practice Guidelines for diagnosis, treatment and follow-up. Ann Oncol. 2013;24(Suppl. 6):vi160-70.
19. Woodruff TK. The oncofertility consortium—addressing fertility in young people with cancer. Nat Rev Clin Oncol. 2010;7(8):466-75.
20. Waimey KE, Duncan FE, Su HI, Smith K, Wallach H, Jona K, et al. Future directions in oncofertility and fertility preservation: a report from the 2011 oncofertility consortium conference. J Adolesc Young Adult Oncol. 2013;2(1):25-30.
21. Kim SS, Donnez J, Barri P, Pellicer A, Patrizio P, Rosenwaks Z, et al. Recommendations for fertility preservation in patients with lymphoma, leukemia, and breast cancer. J Assist Reprod Genet. 2012;29(6):465-8.
22. Klemp JR, Kim SS. Fertility preservation in young women with breast cancer. J Assist Reprod Genet. 2012;29(6):469-72.
23. Jadoul P, Kim SS. Fertility considerations in young women with hematological malignancies. J Assist Reprod Genet. 2012;29(6):479-87.
24. Schmidt KT, Andersen CY. Recommendations for fertility preservation in patients with lymphomas. J Assist Reprod Genet. 2012;29(6):473-7.

25. Coccia PF, Pappo AS, Beaupin L, Borges VF, Borinstein SC, Chugh R, et al. Adolescent and young adult oncology, version 2.2018, NCCN clinical practice guidelines in oncology. J Natl Compr Canc Netw. 2018;16(1):66-97.
26. Fallat ME, Hutter J, American Academy of Pediatrics Committee on Bioethics, American Academy of Pediatrics Section on Hematology/Oncology, American Academy of Pediatrics Section on Surgery. Preservation of fertility in pediatric and adolescent patients with cancer. Pediatrics. 2008;121(5):e1461-69.
27. Gosden R. Cryopreservation: a cold look at technology for fertility preservation. Fertil Steril. 2011;96(2):264-8.
28. Meirow D, Raanani H, Maman E, Paluch-Shimon S, Shapira M, Cohen Y, et al. Tamoxifen co-administration during controlled ovarian hyperstimulation for in vitro fertilization in breast cancer patients increases the safety of fertility-preservation treatment strategies. Fertil Steril. 2014;102(2):488-95.
29. Oktay K, Buyuk E, Libertella N, Akar M, Rosenwaks Z. Fertility preservation in breast cancer patients: a prospective controlled comparison of ovarian stimulation with tamoxifen and letrozole for embryo cryopreservation. J Clin Oncol. 2005;23(19):4347-53.
30. Checa Vizcaíno MA, Corchado AR, Cuadri ME, Comadran MG, Brassesco M, Carreras R. The effects of letrozole on ovarian stimulation for fertility preservation in cancer-affected women. Reprod Biomed Online. 2012;24(6):606-10.
31. Revelli A, Porcu E, Levi Setti PE, Delle Piane L, Merlo DF, Anserini P. Is letrozole needed for controlled ovarian stimulation in patients with estrogen receptor-positive breast cancer? Gynecol Endocrinol. 2013;29(11):993-6.
32. Chung K, Donnez J, Ginsburg E, Meirow D. Emergency IVF versus ovarian tissue cryopreservation: decision making in fertility preservation for female cancer patients. Fertil Steril. 2013;99(6):1534-42.
33. Michaan N, Ben-David G, Ben-Yosef D, Almog B, Many A, Pauzner D, et al. Ovarian stimulation and emergency in vitro fertilization for fertility preservation in cancer patients. Eur J Obstet Gynecol Reprod Biol. 2010;149(2):175-7.
34. Courbiere B, Decanter C, Bringer-Deutsch S, Rives N, Mirallié S, Pech JC, et al. Emergency IVF for embryo freezing to preserve female fertility: a French multicentre cohort study. Hum Reprod. 2013;28(9):2381-8.
35. Cobo A, García-Velasco J, Domingo J, Pellicer A, Remohí J. Elective and onco-fertility preservation: factors related to IVF outcomes. Hum Reprod. 2018;33(12):2222-31.
36. Practice Committees of American Society for Reproductive Medicine, Society for Assisted Reproductive Technology. Mature oocyte cryopreservation: a guideline. Fertil Steril. 2013;99(1):37-43.
37. Massarotti C, Scaruffi P, Lambertini M, Remorgida V, Del Mastro L, Anserini P. State of the art on oocyte cryopreservation in female cancer patients: a critical review of the literature. Cancer Treat Rev. 2017;57:50-7.
38. Levi-Setti PE, Patrizio P, Scaravelli G. Evolution of human oocyte cryopreservation: slow freezing versus vitrification. Curr Opin Endocrinol Diabetes Obes. 2016;23(6):445-50.
39. Gunnala V, Schattman G. Oocyte vitrification for elective fertility preservation: the past, present, and future. Curr Opin Obstet Gynecol. 2017;29(1):59-63.
40. Nitzschke M, Raddatz J, Bohlmann MK, Stute P, Strowitzki T, von Wolff M. GnRH analogs do not protect ovaries from chemotherapy-induced ultrastructural injury in Hodgkin's lymphoma patients. Arch Gynecol Obstet. 2010;282(1):83-8.

41. von Wolff M, Raddatz J, Bohlmann MK, Stute P, Strowitzki T, Nitzschke M. Comments on the letter "Fertility preservation and GnRHa for chemotherapy: debate." Arch Gynecol Obstet. 2010;282(6):717-8.
42. Bedaiwy MA, Abou-Setta AM, Desai N, Hurd W, Starks D, El-Nashar SA, et al. Gonadotropin-releasing hormone analog cotreatment for preservation of ovarian function during gonadotoxic chemotherapy: a systematic review and meta-analysis. Fertil Steril. 2011;95(3):906-14.
43. Kumar P, Sharma A. Gonadotropin-releasing hormone analogs: understanding advantages and limitations. J Hum Reprod Sci. 2014;7(3):170-4.
44. Lambertini M, Horicks F, Del Mastro L, Partridge AH, Demeestere I. Ovarian protection with gonadotropin-releasing hormone agonists during chemotherapy in cancer patients: from biological evidence to clinical application. Cancer Treat Rev. 2019;72:65-77.
45. Blumenfeld Z, Zur H, Dann EJ. Gonadotropin-releasing hormone agonist cotreatment during chemotherapy may increase pregnancy rate in survivors. Oncologist. 2015;20(11):1283-9.
46. Irtan S, Orbach D, Helfre S, Sarnacki S. Ovarian transposition in prepubescent and adolescent girls with cancer. Lancet Oncol. 2013;14(13):e601-8.
47. Practice Committee of American Society for Reproductive Medicine. Ovarian tissue cryopreservation: a committee opinion. Fertil Steril. 2014;101(5):1237-43.
48. Salama M, Woodruff TK. New advances in ovarian autotransplantation to restore fertility in cancer patients. Cancer Metastasis Rev. 2015;34(4):807-22.
49. Wallace WH, Smith AG, Kelsey TW, Edgar AE, Anderson RA. Fertility preservation for girls and young women with cancer: population-based validation of criteria for ovarian tissue cryopreservation. Lancet Oncol. 2014;15(10):1129-36.
50. Abir R, Ben-Aharon I, Garor R, Yaniv I, Ash S, Stemmer SM, et al. Cryopreservation of in vitro matured oocytes in addition to ovarian tissue freezing for fertility preservation in paediatric female cancer patients before and after cancer therapy. Hum Reprod. 2016;31(4):750-62.
51. Rosendahl M, Greve T, Andersen CY. The safety of transplanting cryopreserved ovarian tissue in cancer patients: a review of the literature. J Assist Reprod Genet. 2013;30(1):11-24.
52. Bastings L, Beerendonk CC, Westphal JR, Massuger LF, Kaal SE, van Leeuwen FE, et al. Autotransplantation of cryopreserved ovarian tissue in cancer survivors and the risk of reintroducing malignancy: a systematic review. Hum Reprod Update. 2013;19(5):483-506.
53. Berwanger AL, Finet A, El Hachem H, le Parco S, Hesters L, Grynberg M. New trends in female fertility preservation: in vitro maturation of oocytes. Future Oncol. 2012;8(12):1567-73.
54. Chian RC, Uzelac PS, Nargund G. In vitro maturation of human immature oocytes for fertility preservation. Fertil Steril. 2013;99(5):1173-81.
55. Díaz-García C, Herraiz S. The artificial ovary: any new step is a step forward. Fertil Steril. 2014;101(4):940.
56. Amorim CA, Shikanov A. The artificial ovary: current status and future perspectives. Future Oncol. 2016;12(20):2323-32.
57. Telfer EE, Fauser BC. Important steps towards materializing the dream of developing an artificial ovary. Reprod Biomed Online. 2016;33(3):333-4.

58. Luyckx V, Dolmans MM, Vanacker J, Scalercio SR, Donnez J, Amorim CA. First step in developing a 3D biodegradable fibrin scaffold for an artificial ovary. J Ovarian Res. 2013;6(1):83.
59. Woods DC, White YA, Tilly JL. Purification of oogonial stem cells from adult mouse and human ovaries: an assessment of the literature and a view toward the future. Reprod Sci. 2013;20(1):7-15.
60. Horan CJ, Williams SA. Oocyte stem cells: fact or fantasy? Reproduction. 2017;154(1):R23-35.
61. Truman AM, Tilly JL, Woods DC. Ovarian regeneration: the potential for stem cell contribution in the postnatal ovary to sustained endocrine function. Mol Cell Endocrinol. 2017;445:74-84.
62. Reddy J, Oktay K. Ovarian stimulation and fertility preservation with the use of aromatase inhibitors in women with breast cancer. Fertil Steril. 2012;98:1363-9.
63. van der Kooi A-LLF, Kelsey TW, van den Heuvel-Eibrink MM, Laven JSE, Wallace WHB, Anderson RA. Perinatal complications in female survivors of cancer: a systematic review and meta-analysis. Eur J Cancer. 2019;111:126-37.
64. Hartnett KP, Mertens AC, Kramer MR, Lash TL, Spencer JB, Ward KC, et al. Pregnancy after cancer: does timing of conception affect infant health? Cancer. 2018;124:4401-7.
65. Kenney LB, Cohen LE, Shnorhavorian M, Metzger ML, Lockart B, Hijiya N, et al. Male reproductive health after childhood, adolescent, and young adult cancers: a report from the Children's Oncology Group. J Clin Oncol. 2012;30(27):3408-16.
66. Medrano JV, Andrés MDM, García S, Herraiz S, Vilanova-Pérez T, Goossens E, et al. Basic and clinical approaches for fertility preservation and restoration in cancer patients. Trends Biotechnol. 2018;2:199-215.
67. Vakalopoulos I, Dimou P, Anagnostou I, Zeginiadou T. Impact of cancer and cancer treatment on male fertility. Hormones. 2015;14(4):579-89.
68. Wyns C, Curaba M, Vanabelle B, Van Langendonckt A, Donnez J. Options for fertility preservation in prepubertal boys. Hum Reprod Update. 2010;16(3):312-28.
69. Johnson EK, Finlayson C, Rowell EE, Gosiengfiao Y, Pavone ME, Lockart B, et al. Fertility preservation for pediatric patients: current state and future possibilities. J Urol. 2017;198(1):186-94.
70. Picton HM, Wyns C, Anderson RA, Goossens E, Jahnukainen K, Kliesch S, et al. A European perspective on testicular tissue cryopreservation for fertility preservation in prepubertal and adolescent boys. Hum Reprod. 2015;30(11):2463-75.
71. Goossens E, Jahnukainen K, Mitchell R, van Pelt A, Pennings G, Rives N, et al. Fertility preservation in boys: recent developments and new insights. Hum Reprod Open. 2020;2020(3):hoaa016.
72. Pampanini V, Hassan J, Oliver E, Stukenborg J-B, Damdimopoulou P, Jahnukainen K. Fertility preservation for prepubertal patients at risk of infertility: present status and future perspectives. Horm Res Paediatr. 2020;93(11-12):599-608.
73. WHO. Infertility Prevalence Estimates, 1990–2021. Geneva: World Health Organization; 2023.

Chapter 9

Male Fertility and Cancers

Kuldeep Jain, Bharti Jain, Maansi Jain

■ INTRODUCTION

The last two decades have witnessed an increase in the incidence of neoplasms in children, adolescents, and young adults, especially testicular germ cell tumors (TGCT). Also seen is an increased survival rate in these individuals because of early detection and advances in oncotherapy. Nowadays, more than 75% of young cancer patients are long-term survivors. Both malignancy per se and oncotherapy are detrimental to spermatogenesis. The most common cancers in patients of reproductive age and early childhood are leukemia, Hodgkin's lymphomas, and TGCT **(Fig. 1)**.

It is to be highlighted that even in the absence of commencement of spermarche, testicular development continues. Hence, both chemotherapy and radiotherapy are gonadotoxic to spermatogonial cells.

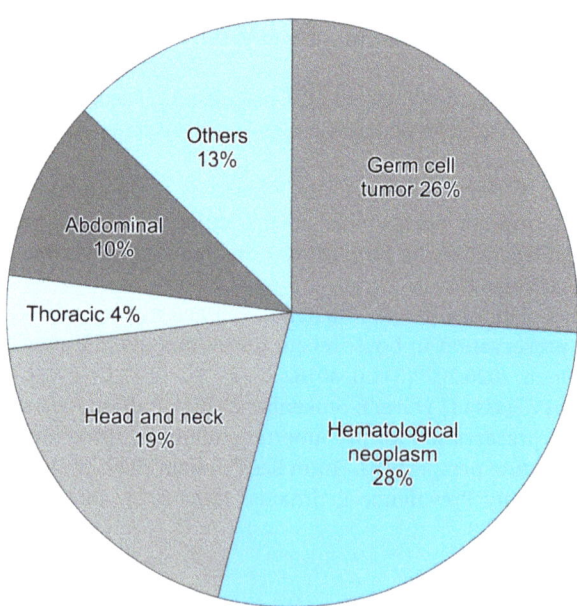

Fig. 1: Most common tumors in male.

Flowchart 1: Effects of cancer on male reproduction.

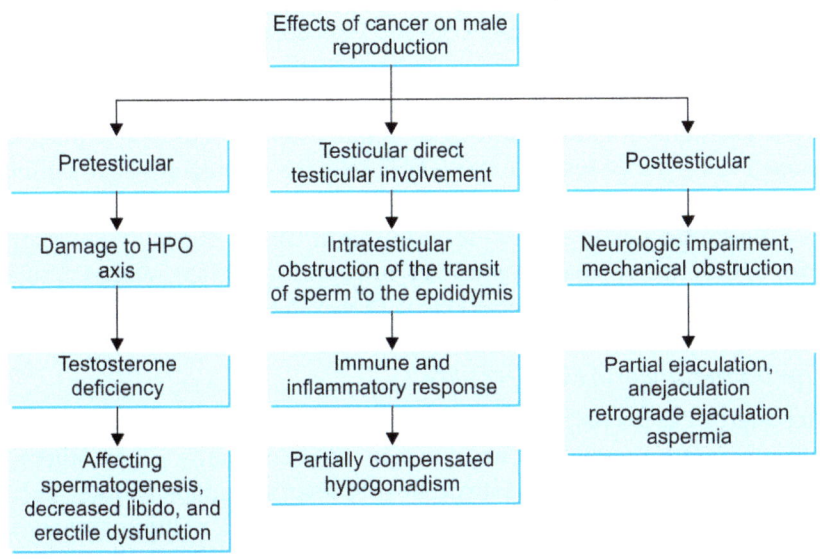

(HPO: hypothalamic–pituitary–gonadal)

DIRECT EFFECT OF CANCER ON MALE FERTILITY (FLOWCHART 1)

Various studies have documented that in malignancies such as testicular carcinoma, leukemia, and lymphoma, semen quality is compromised even prior to gonadotoxic therapy. *Gert R Dohle, in his study* of 764 men referred for sperm freezing prior to chemotherapy, found compromised semen parameters in 64%, especially those with TGCT.[1] In their study, 12% of patients were azoospermic or severely oligoasthenospermic.

Factors Incriminated for Malignancy-induced Infertility

There are multiple factors responsible for low sperm production in malignancies such as radiation-induced damage or direct tumoral invasion of the hypothalamus and the pituitary gland. In leukemia, lymphoma, and central nervous system tumors, there are low level of hormones released by the hypothalamus/pituitary because of stress and downregulation of the hypothalamic–pituitary axis by some tumors, for example, beta human chorionic gonadotropin (β-hCG) produced by TGCT. Associated febrile periods, malnutrition, and deficiencies in vitamins, minerals, and trace elements also hamper sperm production. Systemic inflammatory state with enhanced immune reaction and cytokines released by tumor are also responsible for compromised sperm motility.

Effect of Surgery

Orchiectomy done for primary TGCT and prostate cancer leads to decreased germ cell mass.

Retroperitoneal lymph node dissection, prostatectomy, cystectomy, pelvic exenteration, and low anterior colonic resection induce damage by damaging the ductal system of testis (vas deferens, ejaculatory duct, seminal vesicle).

Cavernous nerve injury or autonomic dysfunction with erectile dysfunction, nerve-sparing modifications, and template retroperitoneal resections can affect erectile and ejaculatory dysfunction.

Chemotherapy and Male Fertility

Prepubertal age is a period when patients are sexually inactive, but testicular development is ongoing. Hence any form of oncotherapy - chemotherapy or radiotherapy is as gonadotoxic in prepubertal gonads as later in life **(Flowchart 2)**.[2] The degree of damage and recovery of spermatogenesis depend on the chemotherapeutic agent and on the total cumulative dose. Alkylating agents such as cyclophosphamide, frequently used in pediatric oncotherapy, induce permanent damage to spermatogenesis with a total cumulative dose of >10 g/m^2. Contrary to earlier beliefs reported in the past, posttreatment gonadal function did not relate to the age at the time of commencement of oncotherapy.

Wallace, in his review, stated that maximum gonadotoxicity was due to nitrogen mustard derivates (busulfan and melphalan) and alkylating drugs (cyclophosphamide and procarbazine). The combination chemotherapy—nitrogen mustard, oncovin (vincristine), procarbazine, and prednisone (MOPP)—regimen given for Hodgkin's disease is very detrimental, resulting in near sterility. However, multidrug regimens applied in young cancer patients, such as Adriamycin, bleomycin, vinblastine, and dacarbazine (ABVD)

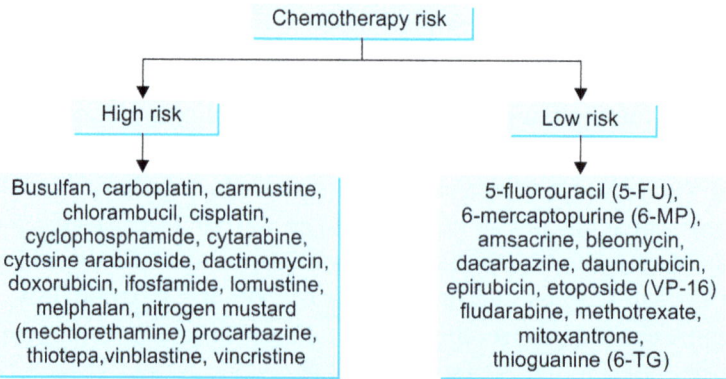

Flowchart 2: Risk of chemotherapy on male fertility.

for Hodgkin's disease and bleomycin, etoposide, and cisplatin (BEP) for TGCT, have a relatively lower risk of permanent infertility.[3,4]

Recovery of spermatogenesis depends on the drugs used and on the cumulative dose given. A major limitation in evaluating the effect of chemotherapy is that new cytotoxic drugs and different treatment protocols are being added. Because of this long-term follow-up, large randomized controlled trials (RCTs) are lacking in literature.

Radiation Therapy and Fertility

Maximum damage by radiation occurs in testicular cancer treated with local radiation within the therapeutic dose range of 16–18 Gy, resulting in permanent damage. Equally higher damage ensues due to whole-body irradiation prior to bone marrow transplantation. In most other conditions, gonadal protecting shields are used **(Flowchart 3)**.

Testicular damage due to radiation depends on the dose and cell type. The seminiferous tubules and germ cells are more sensitive than Leydig cells. In comparison, Leydig cells can tolerate more radiation. The radiation damage to Leydig cells occurs with a dose of >20 Gy, and this dose results in hypogonadism. A dose of 0.1 Gy results in the temporary cessation of spermatogenesis, a dose <1 Gy causes azoospermia lasting 9–18 months, and doses of 2–3 and >6 Gy cause azoospermia lasting 30 months to 5 years to permanent damage. Radiation injury also results in deoxyribonucleic acid (DNA) fragmentation in sperms. Similarly, the recovery of spermatogenesis following radiation is also dependent on doses. The impact of radiation injury to germ cells varies inversely with age. When radiation is given for a prolonged period, it results in increased damage to spermatogonia as sustained injuries hamper the repair and regeneration of reserve stem cell population.

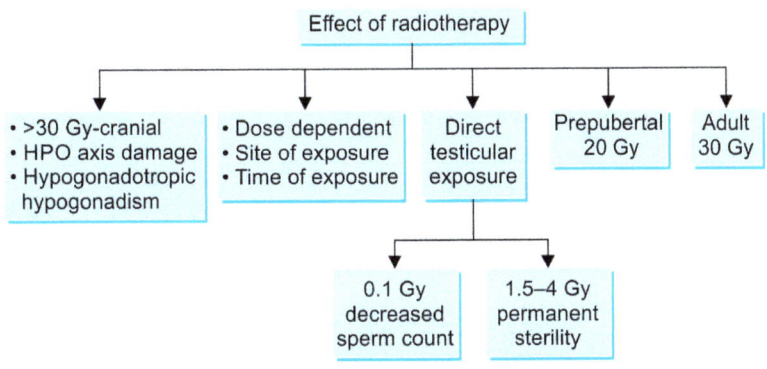

Flowchart 3: Effect of radiotherapy of fertility.

(HPO: hypothalamic–pituitary–gonadal)

Anserini et al., have postulated that with a dose of 0.2, 1, and 10 Gy, spermatogenesis is seen as early as 6 months, 9–18 months, and 4 years, respectively.[5]

■ FERTILITY IN CANCER SURVIVORS

Posttreatment fertility depends on the cancer type, stage, and treatment received, and pretreatment fertility appears to be of prognostic value for future sperm recovery. For instance, in patients who had been treated for TGCT, sperm recovery was high in men with stage 1 seminomas treated with para-aortic irradiation only. Spermatogenesis was seen in 55–80% with cisplatin, and carboplatin-induced damage was even less.[6,7] Procarbazine in the MOPP regimen induces spermatogonial damage, and in patients with Hodgkin's disease receiving more than three courses of MOPP, 85–90% of them had azoospermia for 1 year.

In contrast, of patients receiving the ABVD drug regimen, 90% returned to having normal sperm counts 12 months after therapy.[8] In leukemia, regimens with cyclophosphamide or melphalan are often combined with total body irradiation; this results in permanent sterility in at least 83% of patients.[9] Recovery might take up to 5 years or more to occur. In men with TGCT who received cisplatin-based chemotherapy, normospermia was found in 63% 1 year after chemotherapy; this increased to 80% 5 years after chemotherapy.

■ METHODS OF FERTILITY PRESERVATION

Methods of fertility preservation are shown in **Flowchart 4**.

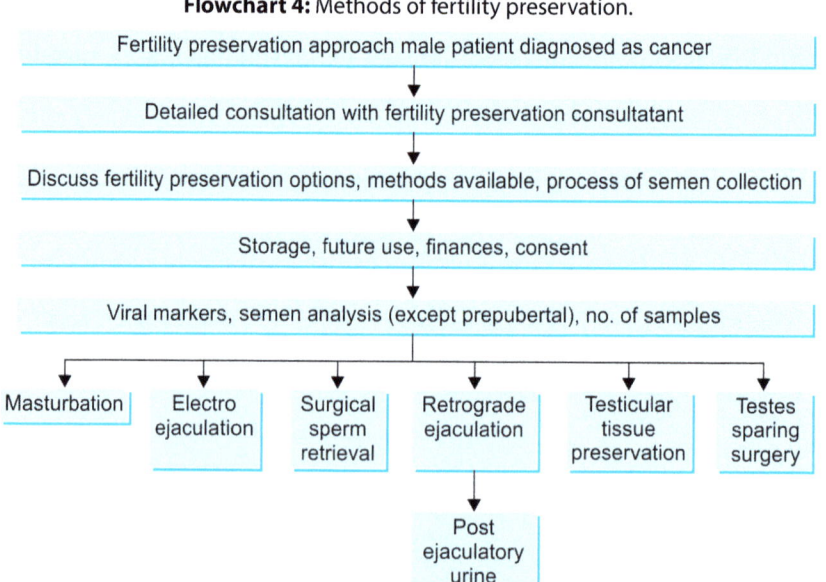

Flowchart 4: Methods of fertility preservation.

Cryopreservation of Spermatozoa
Current Status
In the current clinical scenario, cryopreservation of spermatozoa is the only prevalent and recommended method for fertility preservation in pubertal and postpubertal males. Sometimes, the cryopreserved sample can be used only by assisted reproductive technology (ART) techniques. Literature reviews document the success rate of 33-56% with ART procedures using a cryopreserved sample.[10]

Some of the important facts for cryopreservation of sperm are as follows:
- It is difficult to predict the age of spermarche, and semen quality improves with increasing age. It is also a fact that pubertal development is a better predictor of spermarche than age, so it can be offered to adolescents, at least Tanner stage 3.
- Sperms are obtained via masturbation with 2-3 days of abstinence. At least two to three samples should be collected as semen quantity is often reduced in cancer patients. Freezing is optimally done prior to starting oncotherapy so that there is no iatrogenic damage to sperm DNA. In prepubertal males who cannot masturbate because of lack of sexual inexperience but have intact sacral reflex, semen can be obtained via vibrostimulatory electroejaculation. However, in the current practice, electroejaculation in children is not being widely used. In their study, Hovav et al., documented successful electroejaculation in all adolescents (number of patients = 6, age = 15-18 years[11]). But literature review shows absence of large RCTs documenting use of electroejaculation in pubertal boys with cancer.
- In cases of obstructive azoospermia, sperms are retrieved by microsurgical epididymal sperm aspiration (MESA), testicular sperm aspiration (TESA), testicular sperm extraction (TESE), percutaneous epididymal sperm aspiration (PESA), or microscopic testicular sperm extraction (microTESE). Sperms thus obtained can be used immediately or cryopreserved for later use. Even in some cases of nonobstructive azoospermia (NOA), sperms can be retrieved from some areas in which spermatogenesis is present.
- Semen freezing is a simple and established procedure, with 67% of former young cancer patients having successful sperm banking.[12] Another study also shows that only 27% of men diagnosed with malignancy chose semen cryopreservation. The reason behind few patients opting for semen cryopreservation was lack of information. In cases where semen cryopreservation was unsuccessful, it was seen that these patients were of younger age and had higher levels of anxiety. Also, endocrinological evaluation was of no help to identify this group of patients.

- Another issue that needs to be discussed with the patients is that the cryopreserved sample is usually compromised. On average, sperm freezing decreases motility by 31%, morphology by 37%, and mitochondrial activity by 36%.[13,14]

Testicular Tissue Cryopreservation

Two issues need to be addressed prior to testicular tissue cryopreservation (TTC):
1. Effect on the number of spermatogonial cells
2. Transmission of malignant cells

Effect on the Number of Spermatogonial Cells

The literature shows varied results in the number of spermatogonia on prior exposure to oncotherapy. The decrease in spermatogonial cells is more marked with alkylating agents. Stukenborg et al., reported detrimental effect on spermatogonia germ cells by alkylating agents or hydroxyurea prior to TTC.[15] Medrano et al., reported a dose-dependent reduction in spermatogonia cells after exposure to alkylating agents, cytarabine, and asparaginase.[16] On the contrary, no statistically significant reduction in spermatogonia number was found in children who had received other chemotherapeutic agents. Borgström et al., reported that spermatogonial cells were present in testicular tissue after gonadotoxic therapy, especially in high-risk or relapsed acute lymphoblastic leukemia.[17] These results advocate TTC to children with malignancy relapse or poor response to therapy.

The clinical impact of compromise of spermatogonial cells should be discussed with the patient. In cases of severe compromise, we need to resort to in vitro fertilization (IVF)/intracytoplasmic sperm injection (ICSI).

Transmission of Malignant Cells

More importantly, the cryopreserved testicular tissue should be free of contamination by tumoral cells, especially when dealing with malignancies with a high rate of dissemination of malignant cells such as leukemias. It is important to prevent transmission of congenital malformations, hereditary neoplasms, and adverse neonatal outcomes. An RCT reported a rate of malignant cells contamination by malignant cells (lymphoblastic leukemia) to be as high as 30%.[18]

Current status: At present, in humans, the safety of TTC is unestablished as the mature sperms have not been developed from spermatogonial stem cells.

So, the patient should be counseled about the fact that the reproductive safety of immature testicular tissue samples exposed to gonadotoxic therapy is undocumented.

Despite these reassuring data, more studies and longer follow-up are needed to better clarify issues such as the reproductive safety of previously chemotherapy exposed immature testicular tissue and impact of testicular biopsy on pubertal development and reproductive outcomes.

Another hypothetical solution is in vitro maturation of stem cells into spermatogonia and then xenografting to avoid contamination by malignant cells. But the hurdles of recreating testicular microenvironment conducive for resuming meiosis and sperm maturation have to be overcome.

Future prospective: Germ cell transplantation—this can be offered only to solid organ tumors in the future as there is a limitation to perform 100% accurate cell sorting. This has a risk of contamination by malignant cells.

■ RISKS FOR THE OFFSPRING OF CANCER SURVIVORS

Counseling has challenges as we need to discuss about fertility preservation at a time when the patient is facing an emotional crisis. Concern for a biological offspring is seen in many cancer survivors (73%), and this manifests in the posttreatment period. On survey, around 30–40% pleaded ignorant about fertility preservation, risk of gonadotoxicity, and risk of transfer of malignancy to their biological offspring.

Recommendations from ASRM and ASCO advise counseling the patients and/or their parents about the effects of cancer, the treatment options, mode of use, their current status, and the risk of contamination by cancer cells. Also informed consent on the posthumous use of cryopreserved sperms should be taken.

Risk of Congenital Anomalies in the Future Offsprings

Oncotherapy is potentially mutagenic for the germ cells. So, there is a concern about an increased risk of transmission of malignancy and congenital malformations to the biological progeny due to induction of mutations.

Current available data do not report an increased incidence of congenital anomalies in the biological offsprings of cancer survivors.

Also, except for some forms of hereditary cancers, there is no reported increase in juvenile malignancies in the children of men who have received chemotherapy or radiation therapy for cancer in the past. In contrast to the situation in children from female cancer survivors, these children showed no increased risk for obstetric and perinatal problems or decreased birth weight.[19,20] In contrast to these problems seen in children born to offsprings of female cancer survivors, it is to be noted that there is no report/RCT in cases where IVF/ICSI was done. This is of clinical significance as in many cases IVF/ICSI needs to be done in view of detrimental semen quality as a result of malignancy and/or oncotherapy. Hence, this population is at an increased risk of having congenital birth defects and hereditary cancers as there the natural process of biological selection is bypassed with ICSI. But more RCTs and long-term follow-up are required in this regard.

■ CONCLUSION

Oncotherapy has long-term consequences on reproductive potential, and it results in subfertility and sometimes sterility. Hence, counseling of patients and their parents/guardians, if minor, is important prior to commencement of oncotherapy. As of date, cryopreservation of spermatozoa is the currently practiced option with proven success. Even though cryopreservation of semen can be successfully done, sometimes IVF or ICSI may be required. Cryopreservation is not always possible as in some cases, semen is already compromised even without starting oncotherapy as discussed before. Sometimes, there is failure of ejaculation, especially in prepubertal boys who have no sexual experience. In these cases, even stimulation by electroejaculation fails. So, till date, there are no proven successful options to preserve future fertility in prepubertal boys. However, animal research indicates that harvesting testicular stem cells for in vitro maturation and xenografting might be a potential option in the near future.

KEY LEARNING POINTS
- Early detection of cancer, advances in treatment, and increased survival need to be recognized.
- Cancer per se and treatment strategies (chemotherapy, radiotherapy, and surgery) affect fertility in young adults.
- Various fertility cryopreservation methods are available.
- Timely referral before therapy, detailed counseling, and appropriate fertility preservation method should be offered to all patients before gonadotoxic therapy.
- Sperm preservation is the most common method for fertility preservation in male patients.
- There is a need to collect long-term safety data in offspring of cancer survivors and the risk of congenital malformation.

■ REFERENCES

1. Dohle GR. Male infertility in cancer patients: review of the literature. Int J Urol. 2010;17:327-31.
2. Chemes HE. Infancy is not a quiescent period of testicular development. Int J Androl. 2001;24:2-7.
3. van Casteren NJ, van der Linden GHM, Hakvoort-Cammel FGAJ, Hählen K, Dohle GR, van den Heuvel-Eibrink MM. Effect of childhood cancer treatment on fertility markers in adult male long-term survivors. Pediatr Blood Cancer. 2009;52:108-12.
4. Wallace WHB, Anderson RA, Irvine DS. Fertility preservation for young patients with cancer: who is at risk and what can be offered? Lancet Oncol. 2005;6:209-18.

5. Anserini P, Chiodi S, Spinelli S, Costa M, Conte N, Copello F, et al. Semen analysis following allogeneic bone marrow transplantation. Additional data for evidence-based counselling. Bone Marrow Transplant. 2002;30:447-51.
6. Trottmann M, Becker AJ, Stadler T, Straub J, Soljanik I, Schlenker B, et al. Semen quality in men with malignant diseases before and after therapy and the role of cryopreservation. Eur Urol. 2007;52:355-67.
7. Lee SJ, Schover LR, Partridge AH, Patrizio P, Wallace WH, Hagerty K, et al. American Society of Clinical Oncology recommendations on fertility preservation in cancer patients. J Clin Oncol. 2006;24:2917-31.
8. Tal R, Botchan A, Hauser R, Yogev L, Paz G, Yavetz H. Follow-up of sperm concentration and motility in patients with lymphoma. Hum Reprod. 2000;15:1985-8.
9. Jacob A, Barker H, Goodman A, Holmes J. Recovery of spermatogenesis following bone marrow transplantation. Bone Marrow Transplant. 1998;22:277.
10. van Casteren NJ, van Santbrink EJP, van Inzen W, Romijn JC, Dohle GR. Use rate and assisted reproduction technologies outcome of cryopreserved semen from 629 cancer patients. Fertil Steril. 2008;90:2245-50.
11. Hovav Y, Dan-Goor M, Yaffe H, Almagor M. Electroejaculation before chemotherapy in adolescents and young men with cancer. Fertil Steril. 2001;75:811-3.
12. Edge B, Holmes D, Makin G. Sperm banking in adolescent cancer patients. Arch Dis Child. 2006;91:149-52.
13. Moussaoui et al. Testicular tissue cryopreservation for fertility preservatioj in prepubertal and adolescent boys: A 6 year experience from a Swiss multi-center network. Front Paediatr. 2022;(10): DOI 10.3389/fped.2022.909000.
14. Wyns C, Curaba M, Petit S, Vanabelle B, Laurent P, Wese JFX, et al. Management of fertility preservation in prepubertal patients: 5 years' experience at the Catholic University of Louvain. Hum Reprod. 2011;26:737-47.
15. Stukenborg JB, Alves-Lopes JP, Kurek M, Albalushi H, Reda A, Keros V, et al. Spermatogonial quantity in human prepubertal testicular tissue collected for fertility preservation prior to potentially sterilizing therapy. Hum Reprod. 2018;33:1677-83.
16. Medrano JV, Hervás D, Vilanova-Pérez T, Navarro-Gomezlechon A, Goossens E, Pellicer A, et al. Histologic analysis of testes from prepubertal patients treated with chemotherapy associates impaired germ cell counts with cumulative doses of cyclophosphamide, ifosfamide, cytarabine, and asparaginase. Reprod Sci. 2021;28:603-13.
17. Borgström B, Fridström M, Gustafsson B, Ljungman P, Rodriguez-Wallberg KA. A prospective study on the long-term outcome of prepubertal and pubertal boys undergoing testicular biopsy for fertility preservation prior to hematologic stem cell transplantation. Pediatr Blood Cancer. 2020;67:e28507.
18. Akhtar M, Ali MA, Burgess A, Aur RJ. Fine-needle aspiration biopsy (FNAB) diagnosis of testicular involvement in acute lymphoblastic leukemia in children. Diagn Cytopathol. 1991;7:504-7.
19. Ward E, DeSantis C, Robbins A, Kohler B, Jemal A. Childhood and adolescent cancer statistics, 2014. CA Cancer J Clin. 2014;64:83-103.
20. Fosså SD, Magelssen H, Melve K, Jacobsen AB, Langmark F, Skjaerven R. Parenthood in survivors after adulthood cancer and perinatal health in their offspring: a preliminary report. J Natl Cancer Inst Monogr. 2005;34:77-82.

Fertility and Assisted Reproductive Technology in Obesity and Postbariatric Surgery

Sudha Prasad, Shrinkhala Gupta, Saumya Prasad, Shubhda Gupta

■ INTRODUCTION

The World Health Organization (WHO) defines overweight and obesity as abnormal or excessive fat accumulation, which presents a risk to health. A body mass index (BMI) over 25 kg/m² is considered overweight, and over 30 kg/m² is obese. Women with obesity constitute 41.1% of the United States population, and extreme obesity (BMI ≥40 kg/m²) now affects 9.7% of all women. Across the country as a whole, obesity tended to be higher in women (41.88%) compared to men (38.67%), higher in urban regions (44.17%) compared to rural regions (36.08%), and higher among people over 40 years of age (45.81%) compared to those under 40 years of age (34.58%) **(Table 1)**.[1]

■ EFFECTS OF OBESITY ON REPRODUCTION[2]

In addition to cardiometabolic sequelae of obesity, there is proven evidence which demonstrates that male and female obesity/overweight can cause subfertility or subfecundity and, subsequently, infertility.

There are studies showing that incidence of anovulation, oligomenorrhea, hirsutism, and sexual dysfunction is higher in obese patients than in women

TABLE 1: Proposed body mass index in relation to risk of comorbidity for Asian women.

	Body mass index (kg/m²) WHO	Proposed categories for Asian women	Risk of comorbidities
Underweight	<18.5	<18.5	Low (but risk of other clinical problems increased)
Normal	18.5–24.9	18.5–22.9	Average
Overweight	25.0–29.9	≥23	Increased
Obese	≥30	≥25	–
Obese class 1	30–34.9	25–29.9	Moderate
Obese class 2	35–39.9	≥30	Severe
Obese class 3	≥40	–	Very severe[3]

(WHO: World Health Organization)

with normal BMI. Female obesity influences disruption in the hypothalamic-pituitary-gonadal (HPG) axis, causing hyperandrogenism which has deleterious effects on the follicular environment. Such women also have decreased fertility rate, increased requirement of gonadotropins, and very high chances of recurrent implantation failure (RIF)/recurrent pregnancy loss (RPL).

Male obesity may also lead to subfertility due to a disrupted HPG axis causing hypogonadism, increased testicular temperature, impaired physical and molecular structure of sperm, defective sperm maturation in epididymis, decreased sperm quality, and sexual dysfunction in the form of erectile dysfunction (ED).[2]

■ BARIATRIC SURGERY AND OBESITY

Bariatric surgery is indicated for patients between the ages of 18 and 60 years with BMI of ≥40 kg/m^2 or with BMI between 35 and 39.9 kg/m^2 and comorbidities, in whom surgically induced weight loss is expected to improve the disorder, but only if lifestyle changes and pharmacological treatment have been unsuccessful.[2]

Bariatric procedures are usually classified as (**Figs. 1A to C**)[4]:
- Predominantly restrictive—gastric banding and sleeve gastrectomy
- Predominantly malabsorptive—biliopancreatic diversion with or without duodenal switch
- Combination—Roux-en-Y gastric bypass.

Benefits of weight loss surgery include the following:
- Reduced food intake, body weight, blood glucose levels, and rearrangement of intestinal anatomy, leading to increased glucagon-like peptide 1 (GLP-1) and peptide YY
- Regulation of menstrual cycle, increased ovulatory capacity, and improved fertility in anovulatory and obese women (**Table 2**).

In some studies, no difference was seen in semen parameters for up to 18 months after surgery. Although free and total testosterone was restored after surgery, sperm volume decreased post surgery, and 60% patients showed decreased sperm concentration. Hence, semen freezing is recommended prior to surgery (**Table 3**).[5]

■ PRECONCEPTION COUNSELING IN PATIENTS AFTER BARIATRIC SURGERY

A clinical practice guideline by the American College of Obstetricians and Gynecologists (ACOG), American Association of Clinical Endocrinology (AACE), The Obesity Society (TOS), and American Society for Metabolic and Bariatric Surgery (ASMBS) recommends delaying conception for 12-18 months postbariatric surgery. This is due to rapid and significant weight loss, which starts from the 6th month post surgery to 12 months, causing

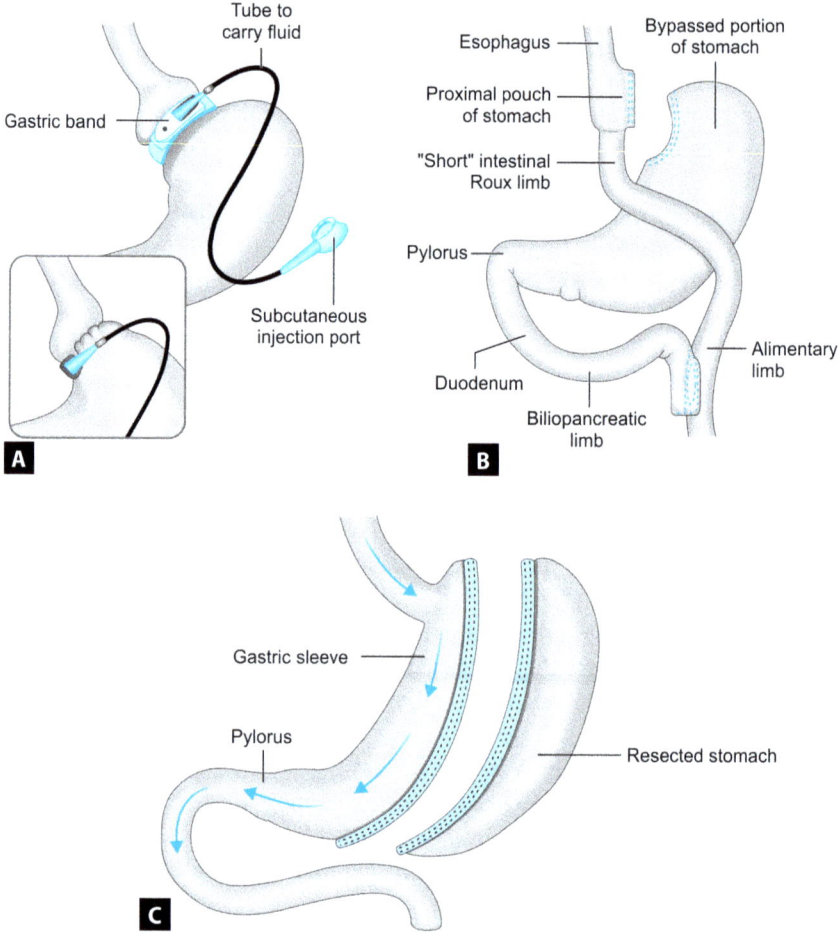

Figs. 1A to C: (A) Gastric banding; (B) Biliopancreatic diversion surgery; (C) Sleeve gastrectomy.
Courtesy: Cornthwaite K, Bahl R, Lenguerrand E, Winter C, Kingdom J, Draycott T. Impacted fetal head at cesarean section: a national survey of practice and training. J Obstet Gynaecol. 2021;41(3):360-66.

severe nutritional inadequacies which can hamper pregnancy. Patients need to be counseled by their clinicians and surgeons that this delay may affect oocyte quantity and quality, which is already decreased in advanced-age women.[6]

Patients should be well informed about the benefit–risk ratio associated with the procedure and the significance of maintaining a healthy lifestyle after the surgery. Moreover, patients who have undergone Roux-en-Y gastric bypass have higher chances of maternal deficiencies of iron, folate, calcium, and vitamins B12 and D. Therefore, reliable contraception is recommended in patients preoperatively, when they begin their very low-energy diet and should be continued in the postoperative phase.[7]

TABLE 2: Effect of bariatric surgery on female fertility.[8]

Different parameters	Outcomes
Bariatric surgery and hypothalamic–pituitary–ovarian axis	Improved sex-hormone profile
Bariatric surgery and PCOS	Weight loss, improved insulin resistance, decreased hirsutism score, menstrual cycle restoration, and ovulation
Bariatric surgery and AMH	AMH normalizes among obese PCOS women
Sexual dysfunction in obese women and effects of bariatric surgery	Female sexual function is resolved after surgical treatment
Bariatric surgery and pregnancy	Reduced GDM, PIH, and macrosomia but increased risk of SGA and prematurity

(AMH: anti-Müllerian hormone; GDM: gestational diabetes mellitus; PCOS: polycystic ovary syndrome; PIH: pregnancy-induced hypertension; SGA: small for gestational age)

TABLE 3: Effect of bariatric surgery on male fertility.[5]

Different parameters	Outcomes
Bariatric surgery and sex hormone	Increased total and free testosterone, reduced estradiol
Seminal outcomes	Volume of semen improved, and viability and count of sperms increased. No response seen on morphology and motility of sperms
Sexual function and satisfaction	Improved sexual quality of life
Bariatric surgery and SHBG	Increased SHBG

(SHBG: sex hormone-binding globulin)

Oral contraceptive pills (OCPs) are the most commonly used method of contraception used by physicians. It offers a failure rate of 5.5% per year in the normal population. This failure is increased in women post surgery due to affected digestive physiology. While patients who have undergone gastric banding are unlikely to have malabsorptive tendencies, women with sleeve gastrectomy and Roux-en-Y bypass will not respond to OCPs.[9]

Banding has less malabsorption syndromes in comparison to sleeve gastrectomy and gastric bypass surgeries. Therefore, it is of utmost importance to rectify any vitamin and mineral deficiencies which are possible in patients who have undergone such surgeries.[9]

Patients need to be counseled about the increased risk of small for gestational age (SGA) fetuses and prematurity after surgery.

CONTROLLED OVARIAN STIMULATION IN PATIENTS AFTER BARIATRIC SURGERY

The ACOG recommends conception postbariatric surgery to be postponed at least 12 months to a maximum of 24 months. It is seen that this time period is sufficient to accommodate the nutritional absorptive malfunctions and hence not have an effect on the subsequent pregnancy of the female.[10]

A national registry study conducted demonstrated less oocyte retrieval rates and embryo freezing rates in comparison to the control group. However, live birth rates between the two were comparable.[11]

Oocytes of obese women are shown to be associated with increased expression of *PGR* and *PTX3* genes in the cumulus cells, which indirectly affects their maturation. Hence, increased doses of gonadotropin for stimulation are required in obese women.[11]

This problem is not encountered post surgery, and patients can be stimulated in an apt fashion without overt high doses of gonadotropins, which are deleterious not only to the oocyte quality but also to the pocket.

Till date, no defined consensus on usage of gonadotropins has been specified for obese patients or for those who have undergone bariatric surgery. Depending on other confounding factors which also have an effect on a patient's fertility, a clinician can use both long gonadotropin-releasing hormone (GnRH) agonist or antagonist protocol. The trigger can be human chorionic gonadotropin (hCG) or agonist when follicles reach above 17 mm on transvaginal sonography (TVS). Oocyte retrieval is to be done 34–36 hours after the maturation trigger.[12]

The important part to keep in mind as a clinician is to not start stimulation before 6–9 months after surgery, nor to delay it so, such that the reserve is diminished altogether.

OBSTETRIC ISSUES IN OBESITY AND POSTBARIATRIC SURGERY[13]

Complications of pregnancy with obesity and its management:
- *First trimester:*[13]
  - First visit at antenatal care (ANC) should comprise weight, height, BMI calculation, and blood pressure (BP) recordings of the patient.
  - Women with BMI >30 kg/m^2 are advised to not gain >7 kg weight in their pregnancy.
  - There are studies which show decreased folate levels and vitamin D3 in obese women. Hence, they should be appropriately compensated for with higher doses of folic acid.
  - Nuchal translucency (NT) measurements transabdominally are difficult due to excessive fat deposition. TVS should be offered to these women.

- Oral glucose tolerance test (OGTT) should be offered to the women on their first visit. If deranged, metformin and insulin should be prescribed.
- Patients should be counseled regarding subsequent comorbidities [such as increased risk of miscarriage, gestational diabetes, preeclampsia, venous thromboembolism (VTE), macrosomia, induced labor, prolonged labor, operative delivery, cesarean birth, postpartum hemorrhage (PPH), and decreased breast milk production] which they may develop due to obesity and one should stay in constant touch with their obstetrician or midwife.

- *Second trimester:*[13]
  - All obese patients should be counseled to undergo an anomaly scan at 18-22 weeks as they are at a higher risk of gross congenital anomaly.
  - Increased chances of gestational hypertension and consequently preeclampsia are seen in the majority of these patients. Such women should have constant BP monitoring using a large-sized cuff (15 × 33 cm) or thigh cuff (18 × 36 cm). Women should be counseled regarding danger signs of impending eclampsia.
  - Repeat OGTT should be advised to women with deranged blood glucose levels at 24-28 weeks.
  - Inaccurate symphysis-fundal height (SFH) measurements are seen in obese women; hence, serial ultrasonography (USG) may be required for constant fetal growth monitoring.
  - Antiobesity drugs are contraindicated in pregnancy. Orlistat is not associated with an increased risk of malformations; however, more evidence is required. Topiramate acts by suppression of appetite but is seen to have increased chances of oral cleft. It is also secreted in milk, posing an unknown risk to the infant. Another drug is lorcaserin which is a serotonin receptor agonist (5HT2c) and acts by appetite reduction. There is no risk seen during embryogenesis; however, it is seen to decrease the birth weight of the fetus in the third trimester.
  - Increased chances of VTE are seen in obese women. All women need to be assessed for the risk of VTE during pregnancy, and LMWH can be prescribed to such patients.

- *Third trimester:*[13]
  - Women should be counseled regarding their higher chances of operative interventions—operative vaginal delivery or lower segment cesarean section (LSCS). They can be offered vaginal birth after cesarean (VBAC) unless there are obstetric contraindications.
  - Obese women undergoing LSCS are at an increased risk of wound infection and thromboembolism.
  - Ultrasound for fetal presentation may be required due to difficulty in palpation of fetal parts per abdominally.

- *Postpartum:*[13]
  - Patients who have undergone LSCS should be allowed mobility as they are at a a higher risk of VTE and bed sores.
  - Breastfeeding should be explained to the patients.
  - Contraception should be advised to all patients. Obesity is a relative contraindication for use of OCPs, and they should be judiciously advised to such patients.
  - They should be motivated to lose weight after delivery, and appropriate nutritional counseling should be offered to such patients.
  - Women who are diagnosed with gestational diabetes mellitus (GDM) should be followed up at 12 weeks after delivery for repeat OGTT.

■ CARE OF PREGNANCY POSTBARIATRIC SURGERY[14]

- Women who have undergone bariatric surgery should wait a minimum of 6–9 months and ideally 12 months to plan their pregnancy.
- This allows for any nutritional deficiencies and malabsorptive symptoms to be resolved before a woman is ready to conceive.
- There is decreased booking weight in patients who have undergone bariatric surgery.
- There are decreased chances of GDM and macrosomia in such patients.
- There is reduced incidence of hypertensive disorders of pregnancy.
- Preconception bariatric surgery is associated with other fetomaternal complications such as:[14]
  - Fetal anomalies: 1.2%
  - Fetal growth restriction: 5%
  - Malnutrition
  - Prolonged labor
  - Increase in chances of induction of labor
  - Postpartum weight retention
  - Juvenile obesity in child
- There was no significant difference found in the incidence of prematurity and premature rupture of membranes between patients who have undergone bariatric surgery versus obese patients.
- There is reduction in fetuses with weight >4,000 g. However, there is an increased incidence of SGA in pregnancies of women who have undergone bariatric surgery.
- The ACOG committee opinion reported increased cesarean section (CS) rates after bariatric surgery, and though this may be due to previous CS, maternal requests, or other obstetric indications, there is still paucity of data regarding the same.
- Nutritional deficiencies are well-recognized complications of bariatric surgery and may lead to reduction in vitamin B, calcium, and fat-soluble

TABLE 4: Obstetric complications following different types of bariatric surgeries.[4]

Obstetrical complications	Gastric banding	Sleeve gastrectomy	Roux-en-Y gastric bypass
Anemia	Low risk	Low risk	High risk
GDM	Low risk		High risk
Surgical complications	Low risk	Low risk	High risk
Birth weight	Increased	Decreased	Decreased
Preterm birth	High risk		Low risk
Gestational weight gain	Increased		Decreased
Booking weight	High	Less	Less

(GDM: gestational diabetes mellitus)

vitamins. The underlying etiology is decreased production of gastric acid, which causes decreased absorption of micronutrients.

- Iron, thiamine, and vitamin A, K, and D deficiencies are common in pregnancies after bariatric surgery. Wernicke encephalopathy and anemia are caused due to deficiency of thiamine and iron. Vitamin D deficiency can lead to bone loss and dental problems in mother and child **(Table 4)**.
- Nutritional deficiencies may also cause fetal malformations and neonatal morbidities such as:[15]
  - Neural tube defects
  - Anemia
  - Preterm birth
  - Cerebral hemorrhage
  - Perinatal death: 1.5%
  - Failure to thrive
  - Deafness
  - Blindness
  - Growth retardation: 5%
  - Epilepsy
- Surgical complications in pregnancy after bariatric surgery:
  - Small bowel obstruction
  - Volvulus
  - Intussusception
  - Gastric band erosion
  - Slipping of gastric band
  - Gastric ulcer
  - Stitch line leak
  - Life-threatening peritonitis.

Early assessment by a senior obstetrician should be done in patients after bariatric surgery, and frequent ultrasound monitoring should be done in women to rule out SGA fetuses. Any abdominal pain should warrant early scanning in collaboration with surgeons. There is no contraindication for vaginal birth other than any obstetric indications.

Perinatal morbidity and mortality are comparable between the different types of surgeries. Complications include risk of neonatal intensive care unit (NICU) admission, decreased APGAR score, congenital anomalies, risk of stillbirth, and perinatal deaths.

There is currently no consensus regarding the type of bariatric surgery regarding women planning a pregnancy. Further studies are needed to demonstrate if restrictive surgeries are better than malabsorptive procedures prior to conception.

■ CONCLUSION

- Bariatric surgery is recommended in patients with BMI ≥40 kg/m^2 or BMI ≥35–39.9 kg/m^2 with comorbidities.
- There are two different types of bariatric surgeries—restrictive and malabsorptive. Malabsorptive surgeries are associated with more complications postsurgery.
- Conception is advised after a minimum of 6 months to a maximum of 12 months. Ovarian stimulation is done by conventional agonist or antagonist protocols.
- There is no statistical difference in live birth rate after bariatric surgery versus obese patients.
- More studies are required for establishment of which surgery is better regarding fertility of the patient and pregnancy outcomes.

KEY LEARNING POINTS
- In females, bariatric surgery leads to an improved ovarian function, regulated menstrual cycle.
- In males, bariatric surgery leads to increased total and free testosterone, sperm counts are increased, there is improvement in semen volume.
- No significant difference in fetomaternal complication as compared to general population in patient undergoing sleeve gastrectomy and gastric banding.

■ REFERENCES

1. Venkatrao M, Nagarathna R, Majumdar V, Patil SS, Rathi S, Nagendra H. Prevalence of obesity in India and its neurological implications: a multifactor analysis of a nationwide cross-sectional study. Ann Neurosci. 2020;27(3-4):153.
2. Kominiarek MA, Smid MC, Lacoursiere Y. Pregnancy in Women with Obesity. Creasy and Resnik's Maternal–Fetal Medicine, 9th edition. Amsterdam: Elsevier Health Sciences Division; 2022. pp. 1166-86.
3. Amiri M, Ramezani Tehrani F. Potential adverse effects of female and male obesity on fertility: a narrative review. Int J Endocrinol Metab. 2020;18(3):e101776.

4. Cornthwaite K, Bahl R, Lenguerrand E, Winter C, Kingdom J, Draycott T. Impacted fetal head at cesarean section: a national survey of practice and training. J Obstet Gynaecol. 2021;41(3):360-66.
5. Moxthe LC, Sauls R, Ruiz M, Stern M, Gonzalvo J, Gray HL. Effects of bariatric surgeries on male and female fertility: a systematic review. J Reprod Infertil. 2020;21(2):71-86.
6. Zaher M, Ali Ahmed B. The male and female patients following bariatric surgery. Assisted Reproduction Techniques: Challenges and Management Options, 2nd edition. Hoboken: John Wiley & Sons, Inc.; 2021. pp. 258-64.
7. Chang YE, Yu TN, Chen CH, Chou SY, Lu BJ, Chen CH. The debated role of bariatric surgery in improving in-vitro fertilization outcomes in morbidly-obese infertile women-a case report and brief overview. Taiwan J Obstet Gynecol. 2021;60:935-7.
8. Micic DD, Toplak H, Micic DD, Polovina SP. Reproductive outcomes after bariatric surgery in women. Cent Eur J Med. 2022;134:56-62.
9. Cheah S, Gao Y, Mo S, Rigas G, Fisher O, Chan DL, et al. Fertility, pregnancy and post partum management after bariatric surgery: a narrative review. Med J Aust. 2022;216(2):96-102.
10. Nilsson-Condori E, Mattsson K, Thurin-Kjellberg A, Hedenbro JL, Friberg B. Outcomes of in-vitro fertilization after bariatric surgery: a national register-based case-control study. Hum Reprod. 2022;37(10):2474-81.
11. Burnik Papler T, Vrtačnik Bokal E, Prosenc Zmrzljak U, Stimpfel M, Laganà AS, Ghezzi F, et al. PGR and PTX3 gene expression in cumulus cells from obese and normal weighting women after administration of long-acting recombinant follicle-stimulating hormone for controlled ovarian stimulation. Arch Gynecol Obstet. 2019;299:863.
12. Grzegorczyk-Martin V, Fréour T, De Bantel Finet A, Bonnet E, Merzouk M, Roset J, et al. IVF outcomes in patients with a history of bariatric surgery: a multicenter retrospective cohort study. Hum Reprod. 2020;35(12):2755-62.
13. Denison FC, Aedla NR, Keag O, Hor K, Reynolds RM, Milne A, et al. Care of women with obesity in pregnancy: Green-top Guideline No. 72. BJOG. 2018;126:e62.
14. Haseeb YA. A review of obstetrical outcomes and complications in pregnant women after bariatric surgery. Sultan Qaboos Univ Med J. 2019;19(4):e284-90.
15. Cornthwaite K, Prajapati C, Lenguerrand E, Knight M, Blencowe N, Johnson A, et al. Pregnancy outcomes following different types of bariatric surgery: a national cohort study. Eur J Obstet Gynecol Reprod Biol. 2021;260:10-7.

Fertility and Assisted Reproductive Technology in Autoimmune Disorders

Bharti Joshi, Varun Dhir

■ INTRODUCTION

The burden of autoimmunity is more prevalent in women as compared to men with peak incidence in reproductive years. This can affect conception as well as pregnancy in terms of increased obstetrical morbidity and mortality. Furthermore, standard treatment regimens may have teratogenic potential and can cause infertility. The care of women with autoimmune diseases like SLE, IBD therefore require a team approach for optimal maternal and neonatal outcome. Meticulous care, preconceptional counseling, disease risk stratification, early recognition and management of complications are the corn stone of successful pregnancy.

■ FERTILITY AND AUTOIMMUNITY

The clinical impact of abnormal autoimmunity on reproductive performance is of prime importance. There is enough evidence saying that female sex hormones play an important role in the etiopathogenesis of many autoimmune disorders. Having said that, autoimmune diseases have predilection for women in their reproductive years. Fertility potential, pregnancy course, and perinatal outcome are affected by these disorders. Previously, these women were discouraged to conceive because of fear of disease aggravation in pregnancy, but over a period, the approach and prospect have changed to a considerable extent. Special emphasis on preconceptional counseling, keeping disease in remission, substituting teratogenic drugs with safe drugs, and close antenatal surveillance help in optimizing perinatal outcome.

▍FERTILITY AND PREGNANCY IN AUTOIMMUNE DISEASE (SYSTEMIC LUPUS ERYTHEMATOSUS, IRRITABLE BOWEL SYNDROME)

Systemic lupus erythematosus (SLE) is a chronic autoimmune disorder having predilection for multiple organs with relapses and remission courses. The various reasons postulated for subfertility in women having SLE are as follows: Suppression of hypothalamic-pituitary axis due to prolonged inflammatory state, antibodies against phospholipids and corpus luteum, diminished ovarian function due to the gonadotoxic chemotherapy and autoimmune oophoritis, renal failure in lupus nephritis, and psychosocial factors. Few studies have also assessed hormonal profile and antral follicle count but failed to give concrete evidence.[1,2] Women with SLE have menstrual irregularities ranging from frequent menses to amenorrhea. Cyclophosphamide therapy may cause premature ovarian failure resulting in amenorrhea and infertility. Those having severe disease exhibit more irregularities and pregnancy-related complications. Impaired reproductive system in these women prevents fertilization or implantation. Available evidence reports a higher rate of disease flare in pregnancy in women having SLE of mild-to-moderate severity. The women having history of past flare, with lupus nephritis and noncompliant to medications, are at an increased risk of disease worsening in pregnancy.

Impaired fertility in males with SLE is attributed to iatrogenic cytotoxic drugs, semen problems, and testicular failure. This is due to the likely damage to seminiferous tubules. Around 40% of males have antisperm antibodies with autoimmune orchitis. Men with SLE are 14 times more likely to have Klinefelter syndrome and, therefore, inability to father a child.[3,4]

The study by Clowse et al. reported a higher risk of preterm labor, preeclampsia, and operative delivery in women with lupus nephritis.[1] A systematic review and meta-analysis reported antiphospholipid (aPL) antibodies and active lupus nephritis as major determinants for maternal complications.[5] The positivity rate for aPL antibodies has been seen in up to 44% of SLE women. Higher disease activity preconceptionally also resulted in an adverse fetal outcome.[6] There is emerging evidence about the serum ferritin, uric acid, estradiol, and uterine artery Doppler as novel predictors of poor pregnancy outcome in SLE women, but before incorporating them into the routine investigation panel, more studies are required.[7]

Women with SLE who have been in remission for the last 6 months have nearly 33% chances of lupus flare. This is similar to SLE women who are not pregnant. Women with active disease at conception may experience flare in up to 60% of cases. Pregnancy complications commonly observed in SLE women are hypertension, preeclampsia, antepartum hemorrhage, preterm labor, postpartum bleeding, and thromboembolic events. The risk of developing preeclampsia is around 15–30% and is seen more in women with underlying renal disease, diabetes mellitus, previous history of hypertension in pregnancy, or who are entering into pregnancy with active disease. Preterm labor is reported more in women taking a high dose of glucocorticoids or immunosuppressive drugs, such as azathioprine, cyclosporine, or having other pregnancy complications. There are increased chances of spontaneous abortion, fetal growth restriction (FGR), and fetal demise reported in various studies. Besides, a higher rate of premature births, congenital anomalies, and increased neonatal intensive care admissions were seen in SLE women.

The risk of developing congenital heart block is around 2% in women with anti-Ro/La antibodies but rises to 20% with previously affected pregnancies. Therefore, close monitoring with fetal echo is required in these women from 16 weeks onward. An entity called "neonatal lupus syndrome" seen in women with anti-Ro/La antibodies is characterized by skin rash, thrombocytopenia, liver function abnormalities, and congenital heart block. Over decades, there is a significant decline in adverse fetal outcomes as a result of better periconceptional care and drugs; still, complications rate remains higher in these women compared to general population. A significant decline in the neonatal lupus is seen in women taking hydroxychloroquine (HCQ) throughout pregnancy.

Irritable bowel syndrome (IBS), a gastrointestinal disorder, affects 20% of the population. An oxidative stress is said to be a possible mediator for subfertility in IBS women. Increased expression of certain inflammatory markers affects the fertility potential; therefore, opting healthy lifestyle and dietary modifications may help to relieve IBS symptoms and its complex effect.

■ PRECONCEPTIONAL CARE AND COUNSELING

Preconceptional counseling is an integral component to optimize perinatal outcome in women with autoimmune diseases such as SLE, scleroderma, or inflammatory bowel disease. They need to be assessed for the various factors that may affect present pregnancy, such as disease activity, concurrent medical issues, organs involved, and coagulation profile. Those having cardiac involvement, interstitial lung disease, and renal insufficiency can have serious maternal–fetal outcomes. The alternatives such as third-party reproduction in terms of surrogacy or adoption should be discussed. Special attention should be given to the previous pregnancy and its outcome in terms of preeclampsia, FGR, stillbirth, or preterm labor. Those having active disease should be advised to defer conception for at least 6 months. Additional laboratory evaluations required in these women are anticardiolipin antibodies, complement levels, and anti-Ro and anti-La, apart from renal and hepatic function tests. These women require multidisciplinary care before conception because of the following major concerns during pregnancy and afterward:

- Risk of maternal disease progression or flare
- Obstetrical concerns in the form of early onset preeclampsia, eclampsia, gestational diabetes, or worsening renal issues
- Adverse fetal outcomes, such as in terms of early trimester pregnancy loss, preterm labor, intrauterine fetal demise, increased neonatal morbidity and mortality, and FGR

- Risk of teratogenicity and adverse events related to chemotherapeutic agents
- Postpartum care and contraception.

ASSISTED REPRODUCTIVE TECHNOLOGY AND AUTOIMMUNE DISEASE

Assisted reproductive technology (ART) is a composite process of oocyte stimulation and retrieval, in vitro fertilization, and embryo transfer in the uterus. The various challenges faced while performing ART in autoimmune diseases include procedure-related problems, medications used before, during, and after ART, and pregnancy-related issues after conception and risk of thromboembolism. Despite extensive use of ART, data on autoimmune diseases is inconclusive. Therefore, the ART procedure should be attempted in SLE women with stable disease after careful selection. Both the European League Against Rheumatism (EULAR) and the American College of Rheumatology have recently issued specific recommendations for ART, pregnancy counseling, and medications for autoimmune disease.[8,9] Counseling should address in detail about ART risks, pregnancy-associated complications along with late-term disability. About one-third of SLE women have aPL and/or anti-Ro/La antibodies which are relevant for ART and pregnancy. Ovarian stimulation causes elevation in the estrogen level and may increase the risk of thrombosis. Therefore, SLE women with aPL antibodies mandate anticoagulation therapy before and after procedure. If they are already on oral anticoagulation, they should be switched to unfractionated heparin which needs to be stopped a few hours before the procedure. There should be proper evaluation for hematological, cardiac, renal, and pulmonary functions because ART risks get aggravated in women with organ dysfunction. Ovarian hyperstimulation in women with renal or cardiac dysfunction may be detrimental and, therefore, should be avoided. Presence of thrombocytopenia, leukopenia, or autoimmune hemolytic anemia may make the procedure complicated. The teratogenic medications such as cyclophosphamide, methotrexate, and warfarin are potentially harmful to gametes and should be replaced months before the planned ART with pregnancy-compatible drugs to know their efficacy and tolerance. Women harboring anti-Ro/La antibodies have a 25% risk of neonatal lupus rash, and 2% can develop congenital heart block, so irrespective of clinical status, these women need to be started on HCQ beginning 3 months before contemplating the ART procedure.

The ART success rate in women with autoimmune disease is often contradictory and derived from small observational studies.[10,11] Some advocate the use of aspirin and steroids to improve the implantation rate; however, this is not supported by high-quality recommendations.[10-17]

The effects of lupus and other autoimmune disease such as inflammatory bowel disease described in the literature do not distinguish between spontaneous and ART pregnancies. SLE women show heterogeneous behavior during pregnancy as few may show quiescence, while others can have flare. Pregnancy in SLE women having aPL, vasculitis, or renal disease usually gets complicated by preeclampsia or renal failure, cardiomyopathy, or cerebrovascular accidents. The primary risk in ART is directly attributed to the maternal disease and multiple gestations-associated issues. Fetal complications in terms of preterm labor, twin-related issues, and neonatal lupus are commonly seen in these SLE women.

If necessary measures are taken, major disease-specific or obstetrical complications can be averted. A multidisciplinary team comprising obstetrician, rheumatologist, and neonatologist should discuss potential complications and associated risks. Women who are severely symptomatic or had an active disease in the last 6 months and have deranged laboratory parameters should be discouraged to conceive. Any prior history of complicated pregnancy, organ dysfunction, or persistence of aPL antibodies is an important predictor of future complications.

■ FUTURE RESEARCH

It is advisable to have national databases for future analysis as information about ART is limited in most of the autoimmune cases. Gathering more information about the effects of medications used to treat these diseases will be helpful for future counseling and knowing aspects of ART and its outcome in these cases.

■ CONCLUSION

Autoimmune diseases like SLE, IBD in pregnancy raises various concerns regarding conception, pregnancy care and its outcome. Meticulous evaluation of the disease parameters, thorough counseling and multidisciplinary approach are the main key components for successful outcome in pregnancy.

KEY LEARNING POINTS

- The burden of autoimmune disorders like SLE, Rheumatoid arthritis, IBD is more prevalent in women of reproductive age group.
- Fertility potential, pregnancy course, and perinatal outcome are affected by these disorders.
- Preconceptional counseling is an integral component to optimize materno-fetal outcome in these disorders.
- The ART success rate in women with autoimmune disease is often contradictory and derived from small observational studies.
- The care of women with autoimmune diseases like SLE, IBD therefore require a team approach for optimal maternal and neonatal outcome.

REFERENCES

1. Clowse ME, Chakravarty E, Costenbader KH, Chambers C, Michaud K. Effects of infertility, pregnancy loss, and patient concerns on family size of women with rheumatoid arthritis and systemic lupus erythematosus. Arthritis Care Res (Hoboken). 2012;64:668-74.
2. Ekblom-Kullberg S, Kautiainen H, Alha P, Helve T, Leirisalo-Repo M, Julkunen H. Reproductive health in women with systemic lupus erythematosus compared to population controls. Scand J Rheumatol. 2009;38:375-80.
3. Carp HJ, Selmi C, Shoenfeld Y. The autoimmune bases of infertility and pregnancy loss. J Autoimmun. 2012;38(2-3):J266-74.
4. Scofield RH, Bruner GR, Namjou B, Kimberly RP, Ramsey-Goldman R, Petri M, et al. Klinefelter's syndrome (47,XXY) in male systemic lupus erythematosus patients: support for the notion of a gene-dose effect from the X chromosome. Arthritis Rheum. 2008;58:2511-7.
5. Bundhun PK, Soogund MZ, Huang F. Impact of systemic lupus erythematosus on maternal and fetal outcomes following pregnancy: a meta-analysis of studies published between years 2001-2016. J Autoimmun. 2017;79:17-27.
6. Jones A, Giles I. Fertility and pregnancy in systemic lupus erythematosus. Indian J Rheumatol. 2016;11(Suppl. 2):S128-34.
7. Stamm B, Barbhaiya M, Siegel C, Lieber S, Lockshin M, Sammaritano L. Infertility in systemic lupus erythematosus: what rheumatologists need to know in a new age of assisted reproductive technology. Lupus Sci Med. 2022;9:e000840.
8. Andreoli L, Bertsias GK, Agmon-Levin N, Brown S, Cervera R, Costedoat-Chalumeau N, et al. EULAR recommendations for women's health and the management of family planning, assisted reproduction, pregnancy and menopause in patients with systemic lupus erythematosus and/or antiphospholipid syndrome. Ann Rheum Dis. 2017;76(3):476-85.
9. Canadian Hydroxychloroquine Study Group. A randomized study of the effect of withdrawing hydroxychloroquine sulfate in systemic lupus erythematosus. N Engl J Med. 1991;324(3):150-4.
10. Eldar-Geva T, Wood C, Lolatgis N, Rombauts L, Kovacs G, Fuscaldo J, et al. Cumulative pregnancy and live birth rates in women with antiphospholipid antibodies undergoing assisted reproduction. Hum Reprod. 1999;14(6):1461-6.
11. Nørgård BM, Larsen MD, Friedman S, Knudsen T, Fedder J. Decreased chance of a live born child in women with rheumatoid arthritis after assisted reproduction treatment: a nationwide cohort study. Ann Rheum Dis. 2019;78(3):328-34.
12. Sills ES, Perloe M, Tucker MJ, Kaplan CR, Palermo GD. Successful ovulation induction, conception, and normal delivery after chronic therapy with etanercept: a recombinant fusion anti-cytokine treatment for rheumatoid arthritis. Am J Reprod Immunol. 2001;46(5):366-8.
13. Chen X, Mo ML, Huang CY, Diao LH, Li GG, Li YY, et al. Association of serum autoantibodies with pregnancy outcome of patients undergoing first IVF/ICSI treatment: a prospective cohort study. J Reprod Immunol. 2017;122:14-20.
14. Geva E, Amit A, Lerner-Geva L, Yaron Y, Daniel Y, Schwartz T, et al. Prednisone and aspirin improve pregnancy rate in patients with reproductive failure and autoimmune antibodies: a prospective study. Am J Reprod Immunol. 2000;43(1):36-40.

15. Taniguchi F. Results of prednisolone given to improve the outcome of in vitro fertilization-embryo transfer in women with antinuclear antibodies. J Reprod Med. 2005;50(6):383-8.
16. Hasegawa I, Yamanoto Y, Suzuki M, Murakawa H, Kurabayashi T, Takakuwa K, et al. Prednisolone plus low-dose aspirin improves the implantation rate in women with autoimmune conditions who are undergoing in vitro fertilization. Fertil Steril. 1998;70(6):1044-8.
17. Sammaritano L, Bermas B, Chakravarty E, Chambers C, Clowse M, Lockshin M, et al. 2019. American College of Rheumatology reproductive health in rheumatic and musculoskeletal diseases guideline. Arthritis Care Res. 2020;72(4).

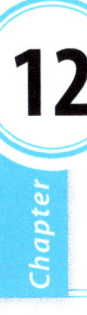

Fertility and Assisted Reproductive Technology in Women on Anticoagulants

Arpita Ray

■ INTRODUCTION

Infertility affects 15–20% of couples. Advanced medical treatment, delaying childbirth, and increasing uptake of fertility preservation for women undergoing cancer treatment caused a gradual increase in demand of artificial reproductive techniques.

It is important to identify the need for thromboprophylaxis in high-risk women who are undergoing controlled ovarian stimulation. It is also important to identify the group of women who are already on anticoagulants and need fertility treatment. They will need a multidisciplinary approach to their treatment involving a hematologist assessing optimum drug suitable while they are going through treatment and embarking on pregnancy, a maternal medicine specialist making these women aware of the risk associated with pregnancy and the impact on the fetus, if any, and a fertility expert addressing the risk associated with in vitro fertilization (IVF) drugs and venous thromboembolism (VTE) risk. Pulmonary embolism of deep vein thrombosis occurs in 0.5–2.2/1,000 deliveries. It depends on the population studied.[1-8]

■ THROMBOPROPHYLAXIS IN PATIENTS UNDERGOING ARTIFICIAL REPRODUCTIVE TREATMENT

There are no definite guidelines or accepted protocols on thromboprophylaxis in relation to IVF treatment. In a recent systematic review,[9] it is shown that the risk of VTE during pregnancy post IVF is double (odds ratio 2.18; 95% CI 1.63–2.92) in comparison to spontaneously conceived pregnancy. It is also noted that there is a very high risk in women who developed ovarian hyperstimulation; it has been noticed that there is up to 100-fold increase in the risk. An absolute risk of 1.7% is noted.

Only evidence-based guideline is issued by the Swedish Association of Obstetrics and Gynecology. This guideline was revised in 2018. They have used grading of recommendations using assessment development and evaluation system while publishing the guideline.

It is important to have a risk assessment system for any woman who is embarking on IVF treatment. The clinician should take a detailed personal and family history of the woman. It is important to have the opinion of a hematologist in high-risk cases. Periconceptional counseling also needs to be mentioned in high-risk cases.

Risk Associated with Anticoagulant Therapy during Pregnancy

It is important to remember the risks associated with anticoagulant therapy to the fetus. Vitamin K antagonists can cause teratogenicity and it is embryotoxic. It is important to discontinue vitamin K antagonist before 6 weeks of gestation. This will avoid the risk of warfarin embryopathy as well as pregnancy loss, fetal bleeding, and neurological developmental issues.[10-12] Any woman who potentially can be pregnant or trying for pregnancy should not take oral direct factor Xa and thrombin inhibitors (e.g., rivaroxaban and apixaban).[13-16]

The embryogenic effect of these drugs is still unknown, and it is best to avoid them.

Fondaparinux[17] has been reported to be used in pregnancy, in patients with severe heparin allergy. However, these reports are in the second trimester or late pregnancy.

Low molecular heparin, unfractionated heparin, and danaparoid (heparinoid) are pregnancy safe and, therefore, can be used in pregnancy for preventative and therapeutic purposes.

However, there are reports of heparin-induced thrombocytopenia and heparin-induced osteopenia. Low molecular heparin has a better safety profile and is widely used in pregnancy.

It should be used cautiously in patients with renal impairment.

Risk Period of a Thromboembolic Episode in Relation to In Vitro Fertilization

This question was addressed in a recent systematic review by Sennström et al.[9] It was seen in six studies[18-23] that, usually, venous thromboembolic events occur within 3–112 days following embryo transfer. A study by Chan and Ginsberg[20] observed a shorter interval (mean 18 days) in the ovarian hyperstimulation syndrome (OHSS) group than without it (mean 57 days). Four studies[20,24-26] showed that the reported gap from embryo transfer to an antepartum thromboembolic episode was between 3 and 28 days.

Risk of Thromboembolism in In Vitro Fertilization Complicated with Ovarian Hyperstimulation Syndrome

A systematic review published by a Swedish group[9] observed that in a study by Rova et al.,[18] women with post-IVF pregnancy who developed OHSS and were hospitalized had a 1.7% increased possibility of a thromboembolic episode in the first 12 weeks. There was a 100-fold increase in risk than background non-IVF population.[18] Hansen et al. showed that there is a 14-fold increase in the risk of VTE when high-risk cases (women with polycystic ovarian disease are a major risk factor for OHSS) were excluded and compared with non-IVF pregnant population.[27]

Recommendations from the Swedish Association of Obstetrics and Gynecology[28,29]

Management of IVF patients and risk assessment for thromboprophylaxis:
- There is no need for routine thromboprophylaxis in patients without any risk factors.
- Patients with OHSS and pregnancy should continue with thromboprophylaxis at least until 16 weeks of pregnancy. Individual organizations should have their individual risk scoring system for risk assessments. We have added the Hem-ARG guidelines scoring system **(Table 1)**.
- Thromboprophylaxis should be continued at least until 4 weeks after the resolution of ovarian hyperstimulation if the pregnancy test is negative.
- Preconceptional counseling and discussion about thromboprophylaxis to be offered if the risk score is >2 **(Table 1)**.
- If any patient needs thromboprophylaxis during pregnancy, then that should be initiated at the beginning of controlled superovulation with recombinant follicle-stimulating hormone (FSH)/human menopausal gonadotropin (HMG)/biosimilar products and estrogen supplementation.
- Scheduling of cycle with combined contraceptive pills or estrogen supplementation should be avoided in patients who need thromboprophylaxis.
- Individualized plan to be generated with the help of a hematologist for very high-risk patients during controlled superovulation.
- Thromboprophylaxis is to be stopped 24 hours before egg retrieval and started 24 hours after egg retrieval.
- Frozen embryo transfer should be considered in a natural cycle instead of a medicated cycle. Risk assessment needs to be done as per risk assessment criteria. Once the pregnancy test is positive, the thromboprophylaxis protocol is to be followed in either low dose or high dose based on risk scores.
- ED stocking can be recommended at any point during treatment.
- *1 point:* Thromboprophylaxis not needed.
- *2 points:* Thromboprophylaxis postpartum once daily for at least 7 days, this includes thromboprophylaxis for a transient risk factor.
- *3 points:* Thromboprophylaxis once daily for 6 weeks postpartum.
- *≥4 points:* Thromboprophylaxis once daily throughout pregnancy and at least for 6 weeks postpartum.

TABLE 1: Summation of added risk points decides management according to the condition [thromboprophylaxis and in vitro fertilization (IVF) guideline issued by the Swedish Society of Obstetrics and Gynecology[29]].

1 point	2 points	3 points	4 points	Extremely high risk
Het FV Leiden	Protein S deficiency	Hom FV Leiden	Prior VTE	Mechanical aortic valve
Het prothrombin mutation	Protein C deficiency	Hom pro-thrombin mutation	APS without VTE	Condition warranting continuous thromboprophylaxis
Obesity	Immobilization	More than one thrombophilia defect	OHSS	APS with VTE
Cesarean section				Recurrent VTE
Age > 40 years				Antithrombin deficiency
Preeclampsia/abruption placenta				
Hyperhomocysteinemia				
Inflammatory bowel disease				

(APS: antiphospholipid syndrome with lupus anticoagulant or cardiolipin antibodies; FV: factor V; Het: heterozygote; Hom: homozygote; OHSS: ovarian hyperstimulation syndrome; VTE: venous thromboembolism)

Notes: (1) Obesity [body mass index (BMI) >28 kg/m^2 in early pregnancy] at booking to the antenatal clinic. (2) VTE in a first-degree relative <60 years. (3) Homocysteine >8 µmol/L in pregnancy. (4) Thromboprophylaxis should be provided during the period of strict immobilization or if the patient has a cast. (5) Patients with previous VTE, or APS without VTE, automatically receive 4 points independent of other risk factors. (6) OHSS—high risk during the entire first trimester. (7) Women in this group are classified as at very high risk of VTE, independent of other risk factors. (8) Warfarin, novel oral anticoagulant (NOAC), low-molecular-weight heparin (LMWH). Not including low-dose acetylsalicylic acid (ASA). (9) Risk factors only in the postpartum period.

- "Very high risk" thromboprophylaxis twice daily (=double dose) throughout pregnancy and at least for 12 weeks postpartum **(Table 2)**.

CONCLUSION

Venous thromboembolism risk is associated with IVF treatment. It is important to take detailed personal and family history before starting any fertility treatment. Risk assessment of each case using a scoring system

TABLE 2: Action plan for thromboprophylaxis for patients with conditions entailing a very high risk of thromboembolic complications.

Condition	Thromboprophylaxis
Recurrent VTE, ongoing oral anticoagulation therapy, and possibly patients with sequelae after previous TE	Ongoing oral anticoagulation therapy and possibly patients with sequelae after previous TE. High-dose prophylaxis LMWH is initiated prior to conception or as soon as pregnancy is confirmed and is continued at least until 6 weeks postpartum or until recommencement of previous treatment
Hereditary antithrombin deficiency	High-dose prophylaxis LMWH is initiated prior to conception or as soon as pregnancy is confirmed and is administered according to individual treatment plan. Antithrombin concentrate if complications and at delivery
APS with TE	High-dose prophylaxis LMWH + ASA 75 mg × 1 is initiated prior to conception and continued at least until 12 weeks postpartum
APS without prior TE	Normal dose prophylaxis LMWH + ASA 75 mg × 1 is initiated prior to conception or as soon as pregnancy is confirmed and continued at least until 12 weeks postpartum
Ovarian hyperstimulation syndrome	Normal dose prophylaxis LMWH is given during the entire first trimester and until the resolution of symptoms
Hyperhomocysteinemia	Folic acid 1–5 mg daily and/or vitamin B6 + vitamin B12

(APS: antiphospholipid syndrome; ASA: acetylsalicylic acid; LMWH; low-molecular-weight heparin; TE: thromboembolism; VTE: venous thromboembolism)

helps in identifying high-risk cases. Women with polycystic ovary syndrome (PCOS) should be thoroughly counseled about increased risk of ovarian hyperstimulation and VTE. The risk of antepartum VTE is doubled than control pregnant population and it is due to a 5–10-fold increase in risk during the first trimester. It is also noted that upper extremity VTE is more common after ovarian hyperstimulation; a suggested explanation is the possibility of drainage of inflammatory peritoneal fluid through thoracic ducts.[30,31] However, bigger studies are needed to establish this relationship. Increased estrogen levels during controlled ovarian stimulation may be responsible for hypercoagulability. OHSS patients were found to have increased hemostatic markers in comparison to normal healthy population.[3,32,33] Detailed discussion, multidisciplinary approach, and counseling help to manage the risk and complication effectively. Each fertility unit should have its own evidence-based risk assessment tools and protocol to reduce risk and complication during treatment and promote safe practice.

KEY LEARNING POINTS

- It is important to identify the need for thromboprophylaxis in high-risk women who are undergoing controlled ovarian stimulation.
- Antepartum risk of VTE post IVF is two times higher in comparison to spontaneously conceived pregnancy.
- It is important to have a risk assessment system for any woman who is embarking on IVF treatment.
- It is important to remember the risks associated with anticoagulant therapy to the fetus.
- Venous thromboembolic episode interval was shorter (mean 18 days) in women with OHSS than without OHSS (mean 57 days).
- Patients with OHSS and pregnancy should continue with thromboprophylaxis at least until 16 weeks of pregnancy.
- Thromboprophylaxis should be continued at least until 4 weeks after resolution of ovarian hyperstimulation if the pregnancy test is negative.
- Preconceptional counseling and discussion about thromboprophylaxis to be offered if the risk score is high.

■ REFERENCES

1. Heit JA, Kobbervig CE, James AH, Petterson TM, Bailey KR, Melton 3rd LJ. Trends in the incidence of venous thromboembolism during pregnancy or postpartum: a 30-year population-based study. Ann Intern Med. 2005;143:697-706.
2. Gherman RB, Goodwin TM, Leung B, Byrne JD, Hethumumi R, Montoro M. Incidence, clinical characteristics, and timing of objectively diagnosed venous thromboembolism during pregnancy. Obstet Gynecol. 1999;94:730-4.
3. Lindqvist P, Dahlback B, Maršál K. Thrombotic risk during pregnancy: a population study. Obstet Gynecol. 1999;94:595-9.
4. Simpson EL, Lawrenson RA, Nightingale AL, Farmer RD. Venous thromboembolism in pregnancy and the puerperium: incidence and additional risk factors from a London perinatal database. Br J Obstet Gynecol. 2001;108:56-60.
5. James A, Jamison MG, Brancazio LR, Myers ER. Venous thromboembolism during pregnancy and the postpartum period: incidence, risk factors, and mortality. Am J Obstet Gynecol. 2006;194:1311-5.
6. Andersen BS, Steffensen FH, Sørensen HT, Nielsen GL, Olsen J. The cumulative incidence of venous thromboembolism during pregnancy and puerperium: an 11 year Danish population-based study of 63,300 pregnancies. Acta Obstet Gynecol Scand. 1998;77:170-3.
7. Jacobsen AF, Skjeldestad FE, Sandset PM. Incidence and risk patterns of venous thromboembolism in pregnancy and puerperium—a register-based case-control study. Am J Obstet Gynecol. 2008;198:233.e1-7.
8. McColl MD, Ramsay JE, Tait RC, Walker ID, McCall F, Conkie JA, et al. Risk factors for pregnancy associated venous thromboembolism. Thromb Haemost. 1997;78:1183-8.
9. Sennström M, Rova K, Hellgren M, Hjertberg R, Nord E, Thurn L, et al. Thromboembolism and in vitro fertilization—a systematic review. Acta Obstet Gynecol Scand. 2017;96:1045-52.

10. Chan WS, Anand S, Ginsberg JS. Anticoagulation of pregnant women with mechanical heart valves: a systematic review of the literature. Arch Intern Med. 2000;160:191-6.
11. Hassouna A, Allam H. Anticoagulation of pregnant women with mechanical heart valve prosthesis: a systematic review of the literature (2000–2009). J Coagul Disord. 2010;2:81-8.
12. Schaefer C, Hannemann D, Meister R, Eléfant E, Paulus W, Vial T, et al. Vitamin K antagonists and pregnancy outcome. A multi-centre prospective study. Thromb Haemost. 2006;95:949-57.
13. Boehringer Ingelheim. (2014). Prescribing information: Pradaxa. Date of text revision: 09/2014. [online] Available from: http://bidocs.boehringer-ingelheim.com/BIWebAccess/ViewServlet.ser?docBase=renetnt&folderPath=Prescribing%20Information/PIs/Pradaxa/Pradaxa.pdf.
14. Janssen Pharmaceuticals. (2014). Prescribing information: Xarelto. Date of text revision: 09/2014. [online] Available from: http://www.xareltohcp.com/sites/default/files/pdf/xarelto_0.pdf.
15. Bristol-Myers Squibb. (2014). Prescribing information: Eliquis. Date of text revision: 08/2014. [online] Available from: http://packageinserts.bms.com/pi/pi_eliquis.pdf. [Last accessed June, 2023].
16. Tang A-W, Greer I. A systematic review on the use of new anticoagulants in pregnancy. Obstet Med. 2013;6:64-71.
17. Dempfle CE. Minor transplacental passage of fondaparinux in vivo. N Engl J Med. 2004;350:1914-5.
18. Rova K, Passmark H, Lindqvist PG. Venous thromboembolism in relation to in vitro fertilization: an approach to determining the incidence and increase in risk in successful cycles. Fertil Steril. 2012;97:95-100.
19. Villani M, Dentali F, Colaizzo D, Tiscia GL, Vergura P, Petruccelli T, et al. Pregnancy-related venous thrombosis: comparison between spontaneous and ART conception in an Italian cohort. BMJ Open. 2015;5:e008213.
20. Chan WS, Ginsberg JS. A review of upper extremity deep vein thrombosis in pregnancy: unmasking the 'ART' behind the clot. J Thromb Haemost. 2006;4:1673-7.
21. Chan WS. The 'ART' of thrombosis: a review of arterial and venous thrombosis in assisted reproductive technology. Curr Opin Obstet Gynecol. 2009;21:207-18.
22. Fleming T, Sacks G, Nasser J. Internal jugular vein thrombosis following ovarian hyperstimulation syndrome. Aust N Z J Obstet Gynaecol. 2012;52:87-90.
23. Salomon O, Schiby G, Heiman Z, Avivi K, Sigal C, Levran D, et al. Combined jugular and subclavian vein thrombosis following assisted reproductive technology—new observation. Fertil Steril. 2009;92:620-5.
24. Aboulghar MA, Mansour RT, Serour GI, Amin YM. Moderate ovarian hyperstimulation syndrome complicated by deep cerebrovascular thrombosis. Hum Reprod. 1998;13:2088-91.
25. Girolami A, Scandellari R, Tezza F, Paternoster D, Girolami B. Arterial thrombosis in young women after ovarian stimulation: case report and review of the literature. J Thromb Thrombolysis. 2007;24:169-74.
26. Kodama H, Fukuda J, Karube H, Matsui T, Shimizu Y, Tanaka T. Characteristics of blood hemostatic markers in a patient with ovarian hyperstimulation syndrome who actually developed thromboembolism. Fertil Steril. 1995;64:1207-9.

27. Hansen AT, Kesmodel US, Juul S, Hvas AM. Increased venous thrombosis incidence in pregnancies after in vitro fertilization. Hum Reprod. 2014;29:611-7.
28. Guideline for thromboprophylaxis during in-vitro fertilisation (IVF). [online] Available from: https://www.sfog.se/media/336079/guideline-for-thromboprophylaxis-during-in-vitro-fertilisation-ivf.pdf. [Last accessed June, 2023].
29. Thromboprophylaxis in IVF. [online] Available from: http://www.nfog.org/files/guidelines/NFOG_Guideline_SWE_160116%20Thromboprophylaxis%20in%20IVF.pdf. [Last accessed June, 2023]
30. Gbaguidi X, Janvresse A, Benichou J, Cailleux N, Levesque H, Marie I. Internal jugular vein thrombosis: outcome and risk factors. QJM. 2011;104:209-19.
31. Bauersachs RM, Manolopoulos K, Hoppe I, Arin MJ, Schleushsner E. More on: the 'ART' behind the clot: solving the mystery. J Thromb Haemost. 2007;5:438-9.
32. Hellgren M, Blombäck M. Studies on blood coagulation and fibrinolysis in pregnancy, during delivery and in the puerperium. I. Normal condition. Gynecol Obstet Invest. 1981;12:141-54.
33. Hellgren M. Hemostasis during normal pregnancy and puerperium. Semin Thromb Hemost. 2003;29:125-30.

13

Fertility and Assisted Reproductive Technology in Cardiac Disease

Harpreet Kaur, Rajesh Vijayvergiya

■ INTRODUCTION

Cardiac disease is one of the major causes of maternal death in developed countries and contributes significantly to maternal mortality in developing nations as well.[1,2] With the advancement in diagnosis and treatment options, many women are reaching childbearing age and might consider an option of assisted reproductive technology (ART). As more and more women are opting for childbearing in advanced age, the risk of cardiovascular diseases (CVD), especially myocardial infarction and hypertensive heart disease, increases in them. The risk of myocardial infarction is 30 times higher in women over 40 years of age compared to those at 20 years.[3] The prevalence of metabolic syndrome in premenopausal females, and hence, coronary artery disease (CAD) is on the rise. In a study evaluating CAD in premenopausal women, these women were found to be at an increased risk of chronic medical conditions such as high blood pressure (BP), deranged sugars, obesity, and metabolic syndrome when compared to healthy controls. Also, these premenopausal women with CAD have dyslipidemia and significantly elevated levels of emerging risk factors such as ApoB, ApoB/ApoA1 ratio, hsCRP, lipoprotein(a), uric acid, T_4, fibrinogen, and total leukocyte count compared to controls.[4] Increasingly more women with polycystic ovary syndrome (PCOS) are being diagnosed with metabolic syndrome and are at an increased risk of CAD. It is a leading cause of infertility and also increases the lifetime risk for CVD.[5] As they conceive after fertility treatment, their risk of developing hypertension and diabetes mellitus (DM) is high during pregnancy and in the later years of life.

Changes in the hormonal environment seen in ART patients increase the BP and peripheral vascular resistance. There is a relatively procoagulant state with a shift in thrombolytic–thrombotic balance. ART-conceived pregnancies exhibit an increased adverse event rate for both the mother and the fetus when compared to natural conceptions, including a higher incidence of hypertensive disorders and an increased risk of thromboembolic events during the first trimester. Ovarian hyperstimulation syndrome (OHSS) can cause dramatic hemodynamic changes and an increase in upper body thrombosis. In women with an underlying heart disease, these hemodynamic

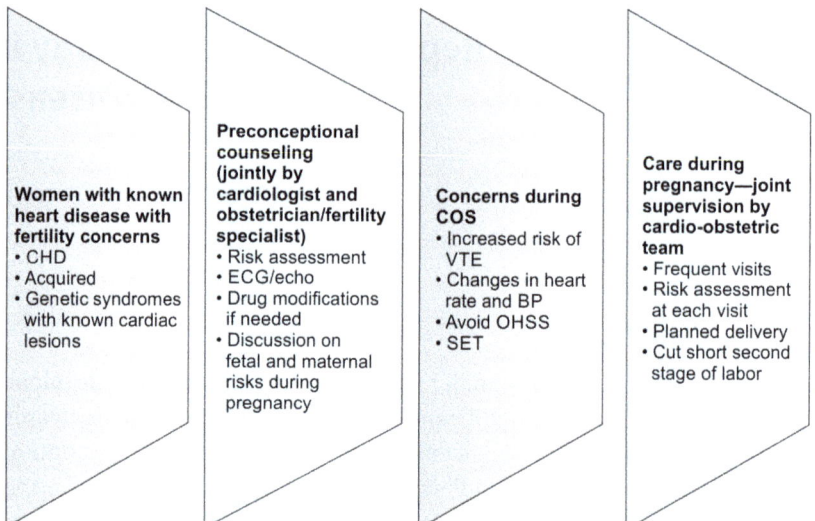

Fig. 1: Algorithm representing fertility and assisted reproductive technology (ART) in women with heart disease. (BP: blood pressure; CHD: congenital heart disease; COS: controlled ovarian stimulation; ECG: electrocardiogram; OHSS: ovarian hyperstimulation syndrome; SET: single embryo transfer; VTE: venous thromboembolism)

changes can have significant effects leading to maternal complications. Prepregnancy risk assessment is essential in identifying women with heart disease who are at a high risk for these complications **(Fig. 1)**.

■ PRECONCEPTIONAL COUNSELING

Women with preexisting heart disease need to be in good health before embarking on pregnancy. They should be evaluated jointly by a team of obstetricians and cardiologists. Any corrective surgery, if required, should be carried out prior to conception.

Pregnancies in Turner syndrome, either spontaneous or those conceived after ovum donation, are at a very high risk for sudden cardiac death mainly due to cardiovascular complications involving aortic root dissection, severe hypertension, or ventricular insufficiency. Women with Turner syndrome undergoing fertility treatment need thorough cardiac evaluation and echocardiography to look for any cardiac lesion, functional status, and thoracic magnetic resonance imaging (MRI) to verify aortic root, cardiac valves, left ventricular function, and hypertension monitoring and treatment.[6] Single embryo transfer should be the preferred strategy in women with Turner syndrome to reduce the risk of cardiovascular complications.[6]

Women with Marfan syndrome need cardiac evaluation and genetic counseling prior to conception. An MRI to look at the aortic root diameter should be done, and the prognosis should be explained accordingly.

Cardiovascular surveillance during pregnancy has to be enhanced, especially in the third trimester and during the peripartum period, to rule out the presence of aortic dissection. Those with cardiac problems should undergo thorough counseling including discussion about the risks to pregnancy and the effect of pregnancy on cardiac disease. Women with a previous history of peripartum cardiomyopathy should be discussed about the increased risk of recurrence in the later part of pregnancy and during the postpartum period.

Women with congenital heart disease (CHD), including cyanotic heart disease, need cardiology evaluation, electrocardiography (ECG), echocardiography, and any correctable surgery if required should be planned in the preconception period. Those with congenital cardiac lesions, especially cyanotic and complex cardiac disease, need to be counseled regarding the risk of CHD transmission to the future child, risk of preterm labor, risk of cardiac complications during pregnancy, and need for hospital admission.

■ CARDIAC DISEASE AND FERTILITY

None of the heart diseases has been found to directly contribute to infertility in both men and women. In the large Danish study on men and women with CHD, it was observed that both men and women with moderate CHD had no increased risk of infertility.[7] While those with complex cardiac disease were more often childless and, hence, showed lower live birth rate (LBR) but once they became parents, they had the same number of children as reference population. Some cardiac conditions such as Fontan circulation have been shown to have impaired fertility.[8,9] Also, menstrual abnormalities and ovulatory defects have been reported in women with complex and cyanotic heart defects.[10,11] Hypoxia is considered to be the main pathological factor in these cases.[9,12] In a recent study on 43 women with complex CHD defects, anti-Müllerian hormone (AMH) levels were found to be low compared to healthy age-matched controls. There was no association between low AMH and saturation levels, which may indicate that low cardiac output is the key pathologic factor for impaired fertility.[11]

Some of the conditions causing infertility such as PCOS might increase a woman's risk of developing CVD and DM later in life. The GRAVID study has shown some unexpected findings about the health of women who had undergone fertility treatment. Those who gave birth after fertility therapy had about half the risk of CVD in the next 10 years compared to women who gave birth without fertility therapy.

■ CONCERNS DURING CONTROLLED OVARIAN STIMULATION

Ovarian stimulation during fertility treatment leads to profound maternal physiological changes.[13] This includes a significant increase in heart rate from pituitary downregulation to peak estradiol levels and a significant decrease in BP from baseline to the luteal phase. There have been concerns about hemodynamic changes during controlled ovarian stimulation (COS), which might affect already compromised heart in women with CVD.

A profound rise in estradiol as a result of ovarian stimulation markedly increases the risk of venous thromboembolism (VTE). This might increase the risk of embolism in women with compromised ejection fraction or with cardiac lesions. Reassessment for VTE risk should be done during ovarian stimulation to determine the need for thromboprophylaxis. In those at high risk of VTE, freeze-all and embryo transfer in subsequent cycles with natural cycle endometrial preparation may be a viable option. All attempts should be made to avoid complications such as OHSS, which can further compromise cardiovascular function due to volume changes and increased VTE risk.

Gestational hypertension and preeclampsia have been found to be increased during in vitro fertilization (IVF) pregnancies which might be correlated with the absence of corpus luteum in hormone-stimulated cycles. Hormone relaxin produced by corpus luteum is normally responsible for relaxation of smooth muscles and dilatation of systemic vascular arteries.[14,15] Pregnancy following IVF is at an increased risk of thromboembolism compared to natural conceptions.[16]

LONG-TERM CARDIOVASCULAR RISKS OF ASSISTED REPRODUCTIVE TECHNOLOGY AND INFERTILITY

Some concerns have been raised regarding the long-term effect of infertility and ART on cardiac status. In the Women's Health Initiative (WHI) study, while evaluating the association of infertility with the incidence of heart failure, it was shown that infertility was independently associated with a future risk of developing heart failure. This risk appeared independent of traditional cardiovascular risk factors and other infertility-related conditions.[17]

None of the studies has shown an increased risk of cardiovascular morbidity in women who had undergone ART. In a retrospective case–control study by Quien et al., no cardiovascular complications or deaths occurred among cases following ART.[18] In a study by Dayan et al., a systematic review of observational studies of fertility therapy, there was no increased risk of developing a cardiac event, but there was a trend toward an increased risk of stroke, and data were inconclusive regarding risks of hypertension and VTE.[19]

CARE DURING PREGNANCY

Women with heart disease should be followed up by both obstetrician and cardiologist. The potential risk factors for the adverse outcomes are poor maternal functional class, significant pulmonary artery hypertension, Eisenmenger syndrome, significant obstructive lesion, heart failure, cyanosis, uncontrolled arrhythmias, and left ventricular systolic dysfunction.[12] Those with cyanotic CHD can have worsening hypoxemia following the increase in right-to-left shunt secondary to decreased systemic vascular resistance. The physiological increase in procoagulant activity during pregnancy can be deleterious in cyanotic patients having hemostatic disorder and hyperviscosity syndrome.[20] The risk of preterm birth, fetal growth restriction, and cardiac events during pregnancy needs to be discussed. In case of CHD, the risk of congenital heart abnormalities in the baby is 3–5%, which is more than the average risk. All women with CHD should be offered a fetal echocardiogram during the second trimester to be done by an accredited fetal medicine/cardiologist. The number of antenatal visits may be more frequent (on an average 2–3 weeks until 20 weeks, 2 weeks till 28 weeks, and weekly thereafter). At each visit, the patient should be asked about breathlessness, palpitations, and exercise intolerance and checked for arrhythmia, BP, and lung bases for pulmonary edema and ankle edema. In cases of cyanotic heart disease, additional investigations such as arterial blood gas analysis may be required as well. In cases of suspected CAD, an electrocardiogram may be done and reveal various findings as well, similar to those who have CVD outside of pregnancy. Fetal well-being should be assessed at each visit including fetal growth and liquor.

A multidisciplinary meeting should be arranged at 32–34 weeks to decide a delivery plan. The general principle of intrapartum management is to minimize cardiovascular stress. This is best achieved by early slow incremental epidural and assisted vaginal delivery. Planned delivery is the preferred approach with a cesarean section reserved for obstetrical indications only. Routinely used oxytocic regimes can lead to major cardiovascular changes; a low-dose oxytocin infusion is probably the safest option.[21] The second stage of labor should be cut short, and a strict intake–output record should be maintained. Infective endocarditis prophylaxis should be given in selected cases.[22]

The management of acute myocardial infarction and its complications should follow the usual principles of care, but fetal considerations may affect the choice of therapy. Management of the patient with CAD and myocardial infarction requires a multidisciplinary approach involving the attending obstetrician, internist, cardiologist, and anesthetist. Ideally, the patient should be treated in an intensive care unit that can provide maternal and fetal monitoring as well as a comprehensive obstetric service.[23] Women with heart disease should be managed in a tertiary care facility high-dependency and intensive care units available.

■ MALE INFERTILITY AND CARDIAC DISEASE

There is no direct association between infertility and heart disease. In the large Danish study on men and women with CHD, it was observed that both men and women with moderate CHD had no increased risk of infertility.[7] While those with complex cardiac disease were more often childless and hence showed lower LBR but once they became parents, they had the same number of children as reference population. Some evidence points to an increased risk of CVD in men with infertility. A recently conducted retrospective cohort study of 13,027 men with infertility showed that those with male factor infertility had a higher risk of developing chronic medical conditions such as ischemic heart disease and DM.[24,25]

■ CONCLUSION

Advancing age, hormonal changes induced by ovarian stimulation, underlying conditions like PCOS and prothrombotic risk of altered hormonal milieu impose a significant cardiovascular risk to women with heart disease undergoing ART. Prepregnancy counseling and a risk assessment by multidisciplinary team is vital before embarking on ART especially in women with complex cardiac lesions and cyanotic heart disease.

KEY LEARNING POINTS

- As more and more women are opting for childbearing in advanced age and undertaking ART, the cardiovascular risks become significant, especially in those with preexisting heart disease.
- Women with known heart disease should be evaluated jointly by a cardiologist and obstetrician/fertility specialty in preconceptional counseling. They should be in optimal health before embarking on pregnancy.
- Patients with Fontan circulation, cyanotic heart disease, or complex cardiac lesions should be counseled about the risks during pregnancy and importance of corrective surgery.
- Management of pregnancy in women with heart disease should be a multidisciplinary management with involvement of obstetrician, cardiologist, and anesthetist.

■ REFERENCES

1. Turnbull A, Tindall VR, Beard RW, Robson G, Dawson IM, Cloake EP, et al. Report on confidential enquiries into maternal deaths in England and Wales 1982-84. Rep Health Soc Subj (London). 1989;34:166.
2. Lewis G. The confidential enquiry into maternal and child health (CEMACH). Saving mothers' lives: reviewing maternal deaths to make motherhood safer 2003-2005. The seventh report on the confidential enquiries into maternal deaths in the UK. Obstet Med. 2008;1(1):54.
3. Cardiac disease and pregnancy (Good Practice No. 13). RCOG.
4. Vijayvergiya R, Kapoor D, Aggarwal A, Sangwan S, Suri V, Dhawan V. Analysis of traditional and emerging risk factors in premenopausal women with coronary artery disease: a pilot-scale study from North India. Mol Cell Biochem. 2017;432:67-78.

5. Scicchitano P, Dentamaro I, Carbonara R, Bulzis G, Dachille A, Caputo P, et al. Cardiovascular risk in women with PCOS. Int J Endocrinol Metab. 2012;10:611-8.
6. Fénichel P, Letur H. Procreation in Turner's syndrome: which recommendations before, during and after pregnancy? Gynecol Obstet Fertil. 2008;36:891-7.
7. Udholm LF, Arendt LH, Knudsen UB, Ramlau-Hansen CH, Hjortdal VE. Congenital heart disease and fertility: a Danish nationwide cohort study including both men and women. J Am Heart Assoc. 2023;12(2):e027409.
8. Cauldwell M, Steer PJ, Bonner S, Asghar O, Swan L, Hodson K, et al. Retrospective UK multicentre study of the pregnancy outcomes of women with a Fontan repair. Heart. 2018;104:401-6.
9. Cauldwell M, Von Klemperer K, Uebing A, Swan L, Steer PJ, Babu-Narayan SV, et al. A cohort study of women with a Fontan circulation undergoing preconception counselling. Heart. 2016;102:534-40.
10. Drenthen W, Hoendermis ES, Moons P, Heida KY, Roos-Hesselink JW, Mulder BJM, et al. Menstrual cycle and its disorders in women with congenital heart disease. Congenit Heart Dis. 2008;3:277-83.
11. Matsushita K, Miyazaki A, Miyake M, Izumi C, Matsutani H, Shimada M, et al. Reduced ovarian function in women with complex congenital heart disease. Int J Cardiol. 2022;7:100317.
12. Siu SC, Sermer M, Colman JM, Alvarez AN, Mercier LA, Morton BC, et al. Prospective multicenter study of pregnancy outcomes in women with heart disease. Circulation. 2001;104:515-21.
13. Fujitake E, Jaspal R, Monasta L, Stampalija T, Lees C. Acute cardiovascular changes in women undergoing in vitro fertilisation (IVF), a systematic review and meta-analysis. Eur J Obstet Gynecol Reprod Biol. 2020;248:245-51.
14. Ginström Ernstad E, Wennerholm UB, Khatibi A, Petzold M, Bergh C. Neonatal and maternal outcome after frozen embryo transfer: increased risks in programmed cycles. Am J Obstet Gynecol. 2019;221:126.e1-18.
15. Von Versen-Hoynck F, Strauch NK, Liu J, Chi YY, Keller-Woods M, Conrad KP, et al. Effect of mode of conception on maternal serum relaxin, creatinine, and sodium concentrations in an infertile population. Reprod Sci. 2019;26:412-9.
16. Henriksson P. Cardiovascular problems associated with IVF therapy. J Intern Med. 2021;289:2-11.
17. Lau ES, Wang D, Roberts M, Taylor CN, Murugappan G, Shadyab AH, et al. Infertility and risk of heart failure in the women's health initiative. J Am Coll Cardiol. 2022;79(16):1594-603.
18. Quien MM, Hausvater A, Maxwell SM, Weinberg CR. Assisted reproductive technology outcomes in women with heart disease. Front Cardiovasc Med. 2022;9:842556.
19. Dayan N, Filion KB, Okano M, Kilmartin C, Reinblatt S, Landry T, et al. Cardiovascular risk following fertility therapy: systematic review and meta-analysis. J Am Coll Cardiol. 2017;70:1203-13.
20. Uebing A, Steer PJ, Yentis SM, Gatzoulis MA. Pregnancy and congenital heart disease. BMJ. 2006;332:401-6.
21. Aggarwal N, Suri V, Kaur H, Chopra S, Rohila M, Vijayvergiya R. Retrospective analysis of outcome of pregnancy in women with congenital heart disease: single-centre experience from North India. Aust N Z J Obstet Gynaecol. 2009;49:376-81.

22. Nishimura RA, Otto CM, Bonow RO, Carabello BA, Erwin 3rd JP, Fleisher LA, et al. 2017 AHA/ACC focused update of the 2014 AHA/ACC guideline for the management of patients with valvular heart disease: a report of the American College of Cardiology/American Heart Association Task Force on clinical practice guidelines. Circulation. 2017;135:e1159.
23. Kealey A. Coronary artery disease and myocardial infarction in pregnancy: a review of epidemiology, diagnosis, and medical and surgical management. Can J Cardiol. 2010;26:185-9.
24. Chen PC, Chen YJ, Yang CC, Lin TT, Huang CC, Chung CH, et al. Male infertility increases the risk of cardiovascular diseases: a nationwide population-based cohort study in Taiwan. World J Mens Health. 2022;40(3):490-500.
25. Eisenberg ML, Li S, Cullen MR, Baker LC. Increased risk of incident chronic medical conditions in infertile men: analysis of United States claims data. Fertil Steril. 2016;105(3):629-36.

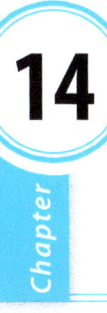

Fertility and Assisted Reproductive Technology in Chronic Renal Disease

Neeta Singh, Garima Patel

■ INTRODUCTION

Globally, chronic kidney disease (CKD) is now recognized as a major health concern.[1] With the Asian population having a relatively higher prevalence, an estimated 17.2% of India's population has CKD, with the disease progressing to stage 3 and beyond in nearly 6% of people,[2] with the prevalence being higher in women than men regardless of age.[3] With a significant decrease in mortality among patients with end-stage renal disease (ESRD) and improvement in their quality of life, many children, adolescents, and young adults are entering into their reproductive age group.[4] Apart from unique and complex physical, psychological, and family challenges faced by this population, they may also suffer from subfertility. Though there are several advancements that have been made in assisted reproductive technology (ART), before undertaking any ART procedures, prepregnancy counseling is a must. This counseling will focus on the degree of renal functional impairment, presence of hypertension, risk assessment for fertility treatment and pregnancy on renal function, a detailed discussion about the outcomes of pregnancy, and, finally, planning the optimal timing of pregnancy.

This chapter focuses on an in-depth discussion of the mechanism of subfertility in patients with CKD, the various aspects of preconceptional counseling, and the necessary modifications to ART protocols for patients in this cohort. Concerning ART complications, additional guidance will be required in these patients. Ovarian hyperstimulation syndrome (OHSS) and multiple pregnancies are two potentially fatal side effects of ART that have been mitigated by recent developments in ART.

■ RENAL DISEASE AND FERTILITY

With the ever-increasing global burden of renal diseases and advances in medical care, the life expectancy of patients with CKD has increased dramatically. Despite the fact that many patients with CKD are now of reproductive age, their fertility and pregnancy rates are significantly lower than those of the general population **(Flowchart 1)**.[5-9]

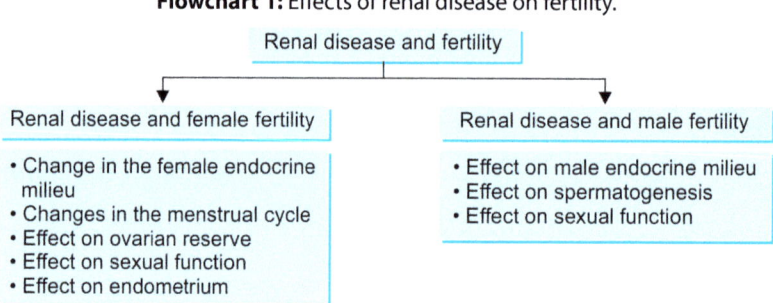

Flowchart 1: Effects of renal disease on fertility.

Effects of Renal Disease on Female Fertility

Up to 92% of women diagnosed with end-stage kidney disease (ESKD) have been reported as infertile.[10] Throughout the stages of CKD, disruptions in female sex hormones and the endocrine milieu result in a progressive loss of fertility.[7] Although an accurate infertility rate among women with CKD is difficult to determine due to poor screening of CKD in the general population of childbearing age, large kidney disease registries can be used to extrapolate this rate.[5] The pregnancy rate in the dialysis population is between 0.7 and 1.1 per 1,000 women, compared to 72.5 per 1,000 women in the general population of Italy, according to a recent study.[11] A similar study in the population of the United Kingdom estimated that the pregnancy rate among dialysis patients was 1.4 per 1,000 women, compared to 79.5 per 1,000 women in the general population.[12,13] Correspondingly, it can be estimated that pregnancy rates in the transplant recipient population are approximately 10% of those in the general population, whereas pregnancy rates in the dialysis population are approximately 1% of those in the general population.[5,11] Despite the fact that the precise mechanism has not yet been deciphered, it is probable that multiple factors are responsible.

Change in the Female Endocrine Milieu

Kidney dysfunction causes female sex hormone dysregulation and disturbance of the hypothalamic–pituitary–ovarian hormone axis.[14-16] This disruption in the distribution of female sex hormones is characterized by an increase in luteinizing hormone (LH) and a decrease in estrogen levels. The absence of pulsatile gonadotropin-releasing hormone (GnRH) release from the hypothalamus leads to impaired LH and follicle-stimulating hormone (FSH) cyclicity and severe hypoestrogenism. This inhibits the surge of LH and prevents the hypothalamus from receiving positive feedback. Anovulation is caused by the absence of cyclicity in circulating gonadotropins and ovarian hormones, in addition to persistent hypoestrogenemia and elevated LH and FSH levels.

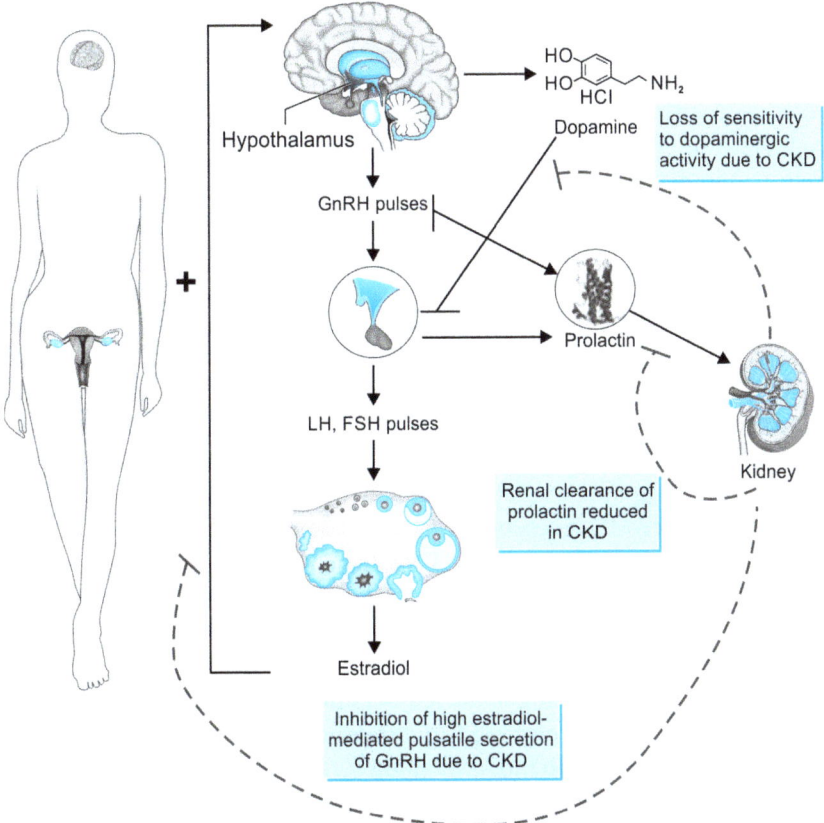

Fig. 1: The hypothalamic–pituitary–ovarian dysfunction in chronic kidney disease (CKD) patients. (FSH: follicle-stimulating hormone; GnRH: gonadotropin-releasing hormone; LH: luteinizing hormone)

Kidney dysfunction reduces the renal clearance of prolactin, thus elevating its levels, further contributing to the anovulation. Due to decreased sensitivity to dopaminergic inhibition, Sievertsen et al., observed an impaired reduction in serum prolactin levels in patients with ESKD after dopamine infusion.[17] The hypothalamic–pituitary–ovarian dysfunction in CKD patients is outlined in **Figure 1**.

Changes in the Menstrual Cycle

A prospective study involving 100 women diagnosed with CKD to determine the prevalence of gynecological disorders in this patient population was conducted.[10] 58% had a menstrual disorder, with uncontrolled menorrhagia being a significant issue that exacerbated the chronic anemia of renal disease; 35% were menopausal.[10] The severity of kidney dysfunction directly impacts the frequency and severity of menstrual disorders. Similarly, in a survey conducted among 129 dialyzed women, 78.7% had regular menses before dialysis, decreasing to 30.6% on dialysis, wherein 43.1% were amenorrheic.[18] Also, on dialysis and after transplantation, 25 and 30.5% of patients suffered from metrorrhagia. However, after kidney transplantation, the menstrual cycle became regular, and fewer were amenorrheic.[18] Thus, this functional state of menopause can be reversed with kidney transplantation or increasing the frequency of hemodialysis (HD).[19]

Effect on Ovarian Reserve

There is a natural decline in female reproductive ability with age. Women are born with a fixed number of eggs, which diminishes with age.[20] This decline in ovarian reserve can be assessed using a hormonal marker. Anti-Müllerian hormone (AMH) is a surrogate marker of the existing follicular pool.[21] A study by Stoumpos et al., found AMH to be 43% lower in women with renal failure when compared to their age-matched controls.[22] However, there was no difference in AMH levels between HD patients and healthy controls.[22,23] Ironically, in women undergoing HD with regular menstrual cycles, AMH was lower than in the control group.[23] This drop in AMH was also observed in those with a renal transplant.[23] Though the exact mechanism is not yet deciphered, the local inflammation due to uremic toxins may influence the ovarian reserve, leading to such a decline in AMH.[22,24] Like all chronic diseases, CKD is also a chronic inflammatory state, with disease activity negatively correlating with the AMH value.[25]

But it is still unclear as to why the AMH values remain unaffected among those undergoing HD. It may result from follicular arrest during the selection of the dominant follicle as a result of complex interactions between AMH and FSH in the hypoestrogenic state of HD.[26,27]

Effect on Sexual Function

Sexual dysfunction is common in women with CKD, with 55% of women on HD reporting difficulty in sexual arousal.[28] There is impaired vaginal lubrication, dyspareunia, and decreased libido among them.[29] In a meta-analysis, an assessment of the prevalence of sexual dysfunction ranged from 30 to 80%.[30] Compared with the general population, women with CKD had a significantly lower overall Female Sexual Function Index (FSFI) score.[30] Though women both on predialysis and on HD had significantly lower desire, arousal, and orgasm scores, those with postrenal transplant retained their sexual function.[31]

Effect on Endometrium

The changes in the menstrual cycle pattern are ill-understood in CKD patients. The relationship between the changes in the endocrine milieu and endometrium morphology is poorly studied. Almost 50% of the women on

HD had atrophia or subatrophia on endometrial biopsy, with proliferative changes in one-third of them. Estradiol concentrations were significantly decreased among those with atrophic endometrial changes, whereas in the rest of the subjects, the increase in serum estradiol was accompanied by a shift in endometrium morphology from the secretion pattern, through proliferative changes to glandular hyperplasia. 75% of the studied population had menstrual disorders, and amenorrhea constituted almost half of them.[16]

Effects of Renal Disease on Male Fertility

Similar to female infertility, the reduction in male reproductive potential is multifactorial and is influenced by a wide range of physiological and pathological factors.

Effect on Male Endocrine Milieu

The endocrine milieu in males with CKD is erratic. The pituitary-gonadal axis is affected only at moderate reduction in glomerular filtration rate (GFR) and worsens progressively as the disease progresses, such that even initiation of dialysis cannot reverse, improve, or normalize the ongoing process. Fortunately, a well-functioning kidney transplant is more likely to restore back this altered endocrine milieu to some extent.[32,33] There are alterations in pulse amplitude and impaired cyclic release of GnRH by the hypothalamus. The serum testosterone concentrations reduce in the presence of elevated serum levels of gonadotropins (LH and FSH).[34] 40-60% of HD patients exhibit hypogonadism,[35] whereas the incidence is lower (15-40%) in those with CKD stages 1-4.[36,37] These elevated levels of gonadotropins may be due to enhanced secretion or a reduced rate of metabolic clearance, indicating poor recovery of spermatogenic function.[34]

Effect on Spermatogenesis

Semen analysis from CKD patients typically shows a low volume of ejaculate, oligozoospermia, or azoospermia with impaired motility. More than 40% of HD patients in a small study had oligospermia or azoospermia.[38] On histopathological examination, decreased spermatogenic activity is observed in all the stages of spermatogenesis, especially in the later hormone-dependent stages. These abnormalities are further deteriorated with the initiation of dialysis therapy. Though occasionally complete aplasia of germinal elements may be present, mostly the number of spermatogonia remains normal with maturation arrest at the primary spermatocytes stage. The severity of cellular depletion is greatest in more mature stages of spermatogenesis.[34] The Sertoli and Leydig cells are normal in number and distribution. The exact cause of spermatogenesis impairment remains unknown. Oxidative stress induced by multiple inflammatory pathways in CKD and exacerbated by the use of glucose-based peritoneal dialysis solutions or the extracorporeal circuit in HD has also been identified as a possible contributor to testicular dysfunction.[39]

Effect on Sexual Function

In CKD stage 5, the prevalence of erectile dysfunction (ED) exceeds 80%.[26] Although the prevalence of ED appears to increase with decreasing GFR, the incidence rate is high for all stages of kidney disease beginning with CKD stage 3.[40] CKD is a contributing factor to the onset of atherosclerotic vascular disease, which in turn affects the penile vascular tree and contributes to the onset of ED. The majority of pathways involved in normal erectile function are affected by testosterone deficiency, including the structure, function, and innervation of smooth muscle cells and the maintenance of the corpus callosum's fibroelasticity. A central testosterone deficiency is a decrease in sexual desire, which plays an important role in ED.[41] Autonomic neuropathy due to type 1 diabetes and uremia, resulting in autonomic nervous system dysfunction, is another possible cause.[42] As CKD-associated ED worsens as GFR declines, it appears plausible that kidney transplantation can ameliorate ED.[30]

■ PRECONCEPTION COUNSELING

Pregnancy is uncommon among dialysis patients, with a very low incidence ranging from 0.9 to 7%.[43] Women with ESRD who wish to become pregnant have the best chance of conceiving if they undergo a kidney transplant because, in some cases, fertility is restored within 6 months of transplantation.[44] Occasionally, however, infertile women with CKD will seek infertility treatment before transplantation "heals" their infertility. This desperation places the nephrologist and infertility clinicians in a difficult position due to the effect of pregnancy or fertility treatment on disease progression and the effect of disease on the outcome of fertility treatment. Also, there is ethical conundrum: Is seeking pregnancy ethically wrong? As the child born to such couples might develop developmental problems in the event of maternal death.[45] According to the Human Fertilisation and Embryology Authority's (HFEA) code of practice, the welfare of the unborn child after fertility treatment must be considered (including the child's need for supportive parenting) prior to the beginning of fertility treatment.[46] The couples should be made aware of the risk-benefit, because certain treatment can be withhold during infertility treatment causing additional risk for the sake of the fetus, thus posing an additional moral dilemma regarding whether women should receive a second transplant if their first transplant deteriorates due to their "voluntary risk-taking" in becoming pregnant.

Optimization of kidney function is a must before embarking on infertility treatment. A multidisciplinary team, including a consultant obstetrician and nephrologist or an expert physician, should conduct a prepregnancy counseling, and only those with stabilized disease activity, controlled on minimized dose of pregnancy-appropriate medications, should be cleared for ART.[47] The associated comorbidities, such as hypertension and diabetes, should be optimized. Drugs such as angiotensin-converting enzyme inhibitors, angiotensin receptor antagonists, or any other teratogenic drugs need to be discontinued and replaced with pregnancy-appropriate medications only after consultation with the nephrologist. Women with known/suspected inherited renal diseases should receive genetic counseling that includes inheritance risk, prognosis, and intervention options such as preimplantation genetic diagnosis.[47] The couples should be informed regarding the increased risk of adverse maternal and perinatal outcomes such as preterm birth, preeclampsia, fetal growth restriction, neonatal unit admission, and increased chance of cesarean delivery to help them make an informed choice.[47]

Effect of Chronic Kidney Disease on Pregnancy Outcome

The degree of renal dysfunction correlates with the risk of a poor pregnancy outcome.[48] Pregnancy-induced blood volume expansion is curtailed by chronic renal insufficiency. They adapt poorly to the gestational increase in renal blood flow, thus accelerating their decline in renal function and leading to a poor pregnancy outcome. The coexistence of maternal hypertension, proteinuria, and recurrent urinary infection may further contribute to the poor obstetric outcome and can be lethal to fetal outcome.[49] Though the pregnancy outcomes of patients with stage 1–2 CKD are acceptable (with the mean gestational age at birth is 38 weeks), those with moderate-to-severe renal damage (CKD stage 3–4) were obviously worse, with an overall live birth rate of only 86.7%.[50] In patients with minimal renal dysfunction, almost 50% were complicated by hypertension, with a perinatal mortality of 50 per 1,000.[51]

Effect of Pregnancy on Chronic Kidney Disease

Numerous previous studies have confirmed that pregnancy has no negative effect on renal function in patients with CKD who have essentially normal renal function. However, it remains debatable whether pregnancy accelerates the decline of renal function in patients with moderate to severe preexisting renal impairment.

Patients with an estimated glomerular filtration rate (eGFR) <40 mL/min/1.73 m^2 and a 24-hour proteinuria >1 g had a significantly increased rate of GFR decline after childbirth, with 30% developing renal failure within 49 months of follow-up.[49] While those pregnant females with mild renal dysfunction (serum creatinine <1.2 mg/dL), minimal proteinuria (<1 g/24 h), and absent or well-controlled hypertension before pregnancy showed that pregnancy had little or no adverse effect on long-term (up to 25 years) renal function.[52] It is not pregnancy per se, but the presence of high serum creatinine and proteinuria are major risk factors for adverse outcomes. In women with chronic hypertension, the risk of delivery before 34 weeks doubles from 20 to 40% in the absence of a gestational fall in serum creatinine that is 10% of prepregnancy values. Overall, it was estimated that pregnancy would bring the need for renal replacement therapy (RRT) forward by 2.5 years. In this cohort, overall RRT rates were low, with only 3% of women beginning dialysis during pregnancy and 7% in the first postpartum year. However, renal replacement was not restricted to women in stages 4 and 5 of CKD.[53] Therefore, planning a pregnancy requires caution and consultation with an obstetrician and nephrologist.

■ PHARMACOLOGY OF ASSISTED CONCEPTION
Clomiphene Citrate

Clomiphene, also known as clomiphene citrate (CC), is an Food and Drug Administration (FDA)-approved selective estrogen receptor modulator (SERM) indicated to treat anovulatory or oligoovulatory infertility to induce ovulation in patients desiring to become pregnant.[54] It induces gonadotropin release by antagonizing hypothalamic estrogens and disrupting feedback mechanisms.

It has been studied in uremic male patients, where it is able to partially correct the majority of gonadal axis hormonal disturbances (improve FSH/LH/testosterone levels).[55] As a result, it is frequently used off-label by men to treat male infertility and secondary hypogonadism due to its ability to increase serum testosterone levels.[56] However, due to the scarcity of similar studies in female CKD patients, it is only hypothesized to correct the female hypothalamic–pituitary–ovarian axis.

Clomiphene citrate is predominantly excreted via the fecal route, with only 8% being eliminated by the kidney. Consequently, no contraindications for renal disease have been reported. The two most adverse effects of CC are OHSS and multiple pregnancy. Though rare, three mild OHSS cases have been reported among 830 ovulation induction cycles with CC.[57] It has long been associated with a multiple pregnancy rate of up to 8–10%, with the majority being twin pregnancies.[58] The recently revised National Institute for Health and Clinical Excellence (NICE) guideline for the management of fertility recommends offering ultrasound monitoring during at least the first cycle of treatment in order to reduce the risk of multiple pregnancy.[59] Therefore, notably, those cycles with multiple mature follicles should be abandoned in CKD females.

Subsequently, females resistant to CC can undergo next line of treatment as proposed by NICE guidelines. It includes either combined treatment with

CC with metformin, laparoscopic ovarian drilling, or gonadotropin therapy. Due to the possibility of lactic acidosis, metformin is contraindicated in women with CKD whose eGFR <30 mL/min/1.73 m^2.[60]

Another alternative oral agent for ovulation induction is letrozole, an aromatase inhibitor. Although it is not FDA-approved, it has several potential benefits over CC, especially for women diagnosed with CKD. These include a higher rate of mono-follicular development, which reduces the risk of multiple pregnancies, the absence of direct antiestrogenic effects on the endometrium or cervical mucus due to the absence of peripheral estrogen blockade, and a lower risk of teratogenicity due to shorter half-life.[61]

Gonadotropins

Follicle-stimulating Hormone and Luteinizing Hormone

Various preparation of both FSH and LH are available, either in single or combination preparations. These are the first-line treatment in patients with hypogonadotropic hypogonadism, hypopituitarism, and those resistant or failed to conceive after several cycles of oral ovulation agents. The most significant adverse effects while using gonadotropins are OHSS and multiple pregnancy. With 10% of these hormones being excreted unchanged by the kidneys, the women with lower GFR and/or creatinine clearance or those with nephrotic syndrome are more susceptible to complications.[62]

Human Chorionic Gonadotropin

Administration of human chorionic gonadotropin (hCG) is crucial to assisted reproduction. During ovarian stimulation in the in vitro fertilization (IVF) cycles, hCG is typically administered as a substitute LH surge to induce the maturation of the oocyte. Additionally, it is used to support the luteal phase following embryo transfer. Approximately 20% of circulating hCG is excreted by the kidneys. The majority of circulating hCG is metabolized by the liver.[63] The effect of severe renal disease on hCG excretion remains unknown,[64] therefore, it is used with caution in such patients.

Gonadotropin-releasing Hormone Agonists

Since the 1980s, GnRH agonists (GnRHa) have been used in ART. By desensitizing pituitary receptors, they inhibit the release of gonadotropins, such as FSH and LH. This phenomenon is known as "down-regulation." A number of metabolic effects, including hypertension, dyslipidemia, and insulin resistance, may result from the use of GnRHa. These side effects are part of a metabolic syndrome that is a risk factor for cardiovascular disease. Patients with renal impairment are cautioned against using these medications.[65]

Gonadotropin-releasing Hormone Antagonists

The introduction of gonadotropin-releasing hormone antagonists, such as ganirelix and cetrorelix, to IVF treatments is relatively recent. They are used over a short period of time, thus reducing drug exposure and the burden of treatment. In addition, triggering with GnRHa in antagonist cycle further diminishes the risk of OHSS. If this protocol is combined with the cryopreservation and subsequent frozen–thawed embryo transfer cycles, the risk of OHSS may be virtually eliminated.[66] These drugs carry a warning for dose modification in mild to moderate renal impairment and are absolutely contraindication in severe renal impairment.[67]

Complications of Assisted Reproductive Technology

Ectopic Pregnancy

Traditionally, ART was believed to increase the risk of ectopic pregnancy compared to the general population, but reported rates range from 0.8 to 8.6% in the ART population.[68] This complication would pose a significant challenge for a woman with ESRD even if detected at an early subclinical stage. Concerns include the possibility of general anesthesia for laparoscopic or open surgical management, hemorrhage before or after surgery, and the complexities of methotrexate-based conservative treatment. Prior to receiving ART, CKD patients should be cautioned regarding this complication.

Ovarian Hyperstimulation Syndrome

The OHSS is a potentially fatal complication characterized by enlarged ovaries (due to follicle enlargement) and an acute shift of protein-rich fluid out of the vascular compartment. OHSS is typically classified as severe when thromboembolic events or respiratory or renal failure are also present. It has been reported that OHSS resulted in obstruction in the transplanted kidney and deterioration of renal function.[69] The pathophysiology of severe OHSS includes an intra-abdominal capillary leak syndrome frequently leading to acute kidney injury (AKI).[70] The significant fluid shifts associated with OHSS would be sufficient to impair any remaining kidney function or threaten the survival of a grafted kidney. The literature is scarce, except few case reports, regarding OHSS or superovulation in women with preexisting CKD.

First-trimester Miscarriage

The spontaneous abortion rate ranged from 12 to 46% among pregnant dialysis patients.[71] Moreover, this is more prevalent among older women and those with other risk elements. Like those associated with diabetes mellitus and hypertension are at particularly high risk for relatively poor pregnancy outcome.[71] The medical management of miscarriage in CKD patients, for whom mifepristone[72] and carboprost[73] are contraindicated, is also a concern.

Multiple Pregnancies

Multiple pregnancies in CKD are like an explosive mix. Twin pregnancy is marked by a more hyperdynamic circulation with greater increase in stroke volume and heart rate resulting from a disproportionate increase in preload in terms of blood volume.[74] This excess volume is burden for the already compromised kidneys. This further compounds the ART pregnancy-related complications such as pregnancy-induced hypertension (PIH), gestational diabetes mellitus (GDM), abruption, chorioamnionitis, and an increased rate of cesarean delivery.[75] Similarly, the presence of CKD, multiple pregnancy, and associated maternal complications compromise the perinatal outcomes of the ART babies. Iatrogenic multiple pregnancies can be prevented in an ART cycle by performing single embryo transfer in women diagnosed with CKD.[47] Therefore, careful prognostication of the subfertile CKD patients is required as it assists helps them in making an informed decision.

Acute Kidney Injury

The AKI has been reported in normal healthy females undergoing ART following compression of ureters by the enlarged bulky ovaries.[76] Also, there have been incidences of AKI following severe OHSS.[70] Intravascular volume depletion, kidney edema due to capillary leakage, intra-abdominal hypertension or compartment syndrome, and obstructive uropathy due to ovarian enlargement are the mechanisms of AKI associated with OHSS.[70] These events can be further compounded in patients with baseline renal insufficiency.

Venous Thromboembolism

Patients undergoing ovarian stimulation with high-dose exogenous gonadotropin administration are at risk for venous thromboembolism (VTE) secondary to supraphysiological hyperestrogenemia and hemoconcentration. This hemoconcentration can also be a part of OHSS spectrum, thus posing a risk for VTE.[77] Fresh embryo transfer in ART is associated with eightfold increase in VTE and pulmonary embolism in first trimester[78] compared to spontaneously conceived pregnancies. This increased risk of VTE is further aggravated in all severities of kidney disease. There is 1.3–2-fold increased risk in mild to moderate kidney impairment whereas ESRD is associated with 2.3-fold increased risk than the general population.[79] Prophylactic or therapeutic treatment with aspirin and low molecular weight heparin is a management of choice.[47]

■ CONCLUSION

From the onset of CKD, fertility treatment and pregnancy pose a challenge. Even when renal function is normal, patients with CKD must undergo rigorous follow-up. Therefore, it creates an ethical dilemma for the infertility specialist, obstetrician, and nephrologist as the patient may seek infertility treatment and pregnancy against medical advice. However, as clinicians, we must recognize that parenthood is the dream of every couple, and we should strive to achieve it while weighing the pros and cons.

KEY LEARNING POINTS
- Kidney disease affects both male and female fertility.
- Optimization of kidney function is prerequisite before starting any fertility treatment.
- Patient should be managed by multidisciplinary team, which includes infertility specialist, consultant obstetrician and nephrologist, or expert physician.
- Vigilance and knowledge of ART complications are required for early recognition and management.

■ REFERENCES

1. Jha V, Garcia-Garcia G, Iseki K, Li Z, Naicker S, Plattner B, et al. Chronic kidney disease: global dimension and perspectives. Lancet. 2013;382(9888):260-72.
2. Singh AK, Farag YMK, Mittal BV, Subramanian KK, Reddy SRK, Acharya VN, et al. Epidemiology and risk factors of chronic kidney disease in India—results from the SEEK (Screening and Early Evaluation of Kidney Disease) study. BMC Nephrol. 2013;14:114.
3. Zhang QL, Rothenbacher D. Prevalence of chronic kidney disease in population-based studies: systematic review. BMC Public Health. 2008;8:117.
4. Foster BJ, Mitsnefes MM, Dahhou M, Zhang X, Laskin BL. Changes in excess mortality from end stage renal disease in the United States from 1995 to 2013. Clin J Am Soc Nephrol. 2018;13(1):91-9.
5. Wiles KS, Nelson-Piercy C, Bramham K. Reproductive health and pregnancy in women with chronic kidney disease. Nat Rev Nephrol. 2018;14(3):165-84.
6. Levidiotis V, Chang S, McDonald S. Pregnancy and maternal outcomes among kidney transplant recipients. J Am Soc Nephrol. 2009;20(11):2433-40.
7. Piccoli GB, Conijn A, Consiglio V, Vasario E, Attini R, Deagostini MC, et al. Pregnancy in dialysis patients: is the evidence strong enough to lead us to change our counseling policy? Clin J Am Soc Nephrol. 2010;5(1):62-71.
8. Lehtihet M, Hylander B. Semen quality in men with chronic kidney disease and its correlation with chronic kidney disease stages. Andrologia. 2015;47(10):1103-8.
9. Holley JL, Schmidt RJ. Changes in fertility and hormone replacement therapy in kidney disease. Adv Chronic Kidney Dis. 2013;20(3):240-5.
10. Cochrane R, Regan L. Undetected gynaecological disorders in women with renal disease. Hum Reprod. 1997;12(4):667-70.
11. Piccoli GB, Cabiddu G, Daidone G, Guzzo G, Maxia S, Ciniglio I, et al. The children of dialysis: live-born babies from on-dialysis mothers in Italy—an epidemiological perspective comparing dialysis, kidney transplantation and the overall population. Nephrol Dial Transplant. 2014;29(8):1578-86.
12. Knight M, Kurinczuk JJ, Tuffnell D, Brocklehurst P. The UK Obstetric Surveillance System for rare disorders of pregnancy. BJOG. 2005;112(3):263-5.
13. Office for National Statistics. Conceptions in England and Wales Statistical bulletins. [online] Available from: https://www.ons.gov.uk/peoplepopulation

andcommunity/birthsdeathsandmarriages/conceptionandfertilityrates/ bulletins/conceptionstatistics/previousReleases. [Last accessed June, 2023].
14. Ahmed SB, Ramesh S. Sex hormones in women with kidney disease. Nephrol Dial Transplant. 2016;31(11):1787-95.
15. Holley JL, Schmidt RJ, Bender FH, Dumler F, Schiff M. Gynecologic and reproductive issues in women on dialysis. Am J Kidney Dis. 1997;29(5):685-90.
16. Matuszkiewicz-Rowinska J, Skórzewska K, Radowicki S, Niemczyk S, Sokalski A, Przedlacki J, et al. Endometrial morphology and pituitary-gonadal axis dysfunction in women of reproductive age undergoing chronic haemodialysis—a multicentre study. Nephrol Dial Transplant. 2004;19(8):2074-7.
17. Sievertsen GD, Lim VS, Nakawatase C, Frohman LA. Metabolic clearance and secretion rates of human prolactin in normal subjects and in patients with chronic renal failure. J Clin Endocrinol Metab. 1980;50(5):846-52.
18. Chakhtoura Z, Meunier M, Caby J, Mercadal L, Arzouk N, Barrou B, et al. Gynecologic follow up of 129 women on dialysis and after kidney transplantation: a retrospective cohort study. Eur J Obstet Gynecol Reprod Biol. 2015;187:1-5.
19. Pietrzak B, Wielgos M, Kaminski P, Jabiry-Zieniewicz Z, Bobrowska K. Menstrual cycle and sex hormone profile in kidney-transplanted women. Neuro Endocrinol Lett. 2006;27(1-2):198-202.
20. Cleveland Clinic. Female Reproductive System: Structure & Function. [online] Available from: https://my.clevelandclinic.org/health/articles/9118-female-reproductive-system. [Last accessed June, 2023].
21. Moolhuijsen LME, Visser JA. Anti-Müllerian hormone and ovarian reserve: update on assessing ovarian function. J Clin Endocrinol Metab. 2020;105(11):dgaa513.
22. Stoumpos S, Lees J, Welsh P, Hund M, Geddes CC, Nelson SM, et al. The utility of anti-Müllerian hormone in women with chronic kidney disease, on haemodialysis and after kidney transplantation. Reprod Biomed Online. 2018;36(2):219-26.
23. Sikora-Grabka E, Adamczak M, Kuczera P, Szotowska M, Madej P, Wiecek A. Serum anti-Müllerian hormone concentration in young women with chronic kidney disease on hemodialysis, and after successful kidney transplantation. Kidney Blood Press Res. 2016;41(5):552-60.
24. Cui L, Sheng Y, Sun M, Hu J, Qin Y, Chen ZJ. Chronic pelvic inflammation diminished ovarian reserve as indicated by serum anti Müllerian hormone. PLoS One. 2016;11(6):e0156130.
25. Şenateş E, Çolak Y, Erdem ED, Yeşil A, Coşkunpınar E, Şahin Ö, et al. Serum anti-Müllerian hormone levels are lower in reproductive-age women with Crohn's disease compared to healthy control women. J Crohns Colitis. 2013;7(2):e29-34.
26. Dumont A, Robin G, Catteau-Jonard S, Dewailly D. Role of anti-Müllerian hormone in pathophysiology, diagnosis and treatment of polycystic ovary syndrome: a review. Reprod Biol Endocrinol. 2015;13:137.
27. Garg D, Tal R. The role of AMH in the pathophysiology of polycystic ovarian syndrome. Reprod BioMed Online. 2016;33(1):15-28.
28. Pigny P, Merlen E, Robert Y, Cortet-Rudelli C, Decanter C, Jonard S, et al. Elevated serum level of anti-mullerian hormone in patients with polycystic ovary syndrome: relationship to the ovarian follicle excess and to the follicular arrest. J Clin Endocrinol Metab. 2003;88(12):5957-62.
29. Bellinghieri G, Santoro D, Mallamace A, Savica V. Sexual dysfunction in chronic renal failure. J Nephrol. 2008;21(Suppl. 13):S113-7.

30. Navaneethan SD, Vecchio M, Johnson DW, Saglimbene V, Graziano G, Pellegrini F, et al. Prevalence and correlates of self-reported sexual dysfunction in CKD: a meta-analysis of observational studies. Am J Kidney Dis. 2010;56(4):670-85.
31. Basok EK, Atsu N, Rifaioglu MM, Kantarci G, Yildirim A, Tokuc R. Assessment of female sexual function and quality of life in predialysis, peritoneal dialysis, hemodialysis, and renal transplant patients. Int Urol Nephrol. 2009;41(3):473-81.
32. Holdsworth SR, de Kretser DM, Atkins RC. A comparison of hemodialysis and transplantation in reversing the uremic disturbance of male reproductive function. Clin Nephrol. 1978;10(4):146-50.
33. Diemont WL, Vruggink PA, Meuleman EJ, Doesburg WH, Lemmens WA, Berden JH. Sexual dysfunction after renal replacement therapy. Am J Kidney Dis. 2000;35(5):845-51.
34. Handelsman DJ. Hypothalamic-pituitary gonadal dysfunction in renal failure, dialysis and renal transplantation. Endocr Rev. 1985;6(2):151-82.
35. Kyriazis J, Tzanakis I, Stylianou K, Katsipi I, Moisiadis D, Papadaki A, et al. Low serum testosterone, arterial stiffness and mortality in male haemodialysis patients. Nephrol Dial Transplant. 2011;26(9):2971-7.
36. Gungor O, Kircelli F, Carrero JJ, Asci G, Toz H, Tatar E, et al. Endogenous testosterone and mortality in male hemodialysis patients: is it the result of aging? Clin J Am Soc Nephrol. 2010;5(11):2018-23.
37. Yilmaz MI, Sonmez A, Qureshi AR, Saglam M, Stenvinkel P, Yaman H, et al. Endogenous testosterone, endothelial dysfunction, and cardiovascular events in men with nondialysis chronic kidney disease. Clin J Am Soc Nephrol. 2011;6(7):1617-25.
38. Prem AR, Punekar SV, Kalpana M, Kelkar AR, Acharya VN. Male reproductive function in uraemia: efficacy of haemodialysis and renal transplantation. Br J Urol. 1996;78(4):635-8.
39. Shiraishi K, Shimabukuro T, Naito K. Effects of hemodialysis on testicular volume and oxidative stress in humans. J Urol. 2008;180(2):644-50.
40. Rosas SE, Joffe M, Franklin E, Strom BL, Kotzker W, Brensinger C, et al. Prevalence and determinants of erectile dysfunction in hemodialysis patients. Kidney Int. 2001;59(6):2259-66.
41. Isidori AM, Buvat J, Corona G, Goldstein I, Jannini EA, Lenzi A, et al. A critical analysis of the role of testosterone in erectile function: from pathophysiology to treatment—a systematic review. Eur Urol. 2014;65(1):99-112.
42. Vita G, Bellinghieri G, Trusso A, Costantino G, Santoro D, Monteleone F, et al. Uremic autonomic neuropathy studied by spectral analysis of heart rate. Kidney Int. 1999;56(1):232-7.
43. Shah S, Verma P. Overview of pregnancy in renal transplant patients. Int J Nephrol. 2016;2016:4539342.
44. Saha MT, Saha HHT, Niskanen LK, Salmela KT, Pasternack AI. Time course of serum prolactin and sex hormones following successful renal transplantation. Nephron. 2002;92(3):735-7.
45. Marks NF, Jun H, Song J. Death of parents and adult psychological and physical well-being: a prospective U.S. National Study. J Fam Issues. 2007;28(12):1611-38.
46. Human Fertilisation & Embryology Authority. The new version of the Code of Practice is now available. [online] Available from: https://www.hfea.gov. uk/about-us/news-and-press-releases/2019-news-and-press-releases/

new-version-of-the-code-of-practice-has-been-launched/. [Last accessed June, 2023].
47. Wiles K, Chappell L, Clark K, Elman L, Hall M, Lightstone L, et al. Clinical practice guideline on pregnancy and renal disease. BMC Nephrol. 2019;20(1):401.
48. Jungers P, Chauveau D, Choukroun G, Moynot A, Skhiri H, Houillier P, et al. Pregnancy in women with impaired renal function. Clin Nephrol. 1997;47(5):281-8.
49. Imbasciati E, Gregorini G, Cabiddu G, Gammaro L, Ambroso G, Del Giudice A, et al. Pregnancy in CKD stages 3 to 5: fetal and maternal outcomes. Am J Kidney Dis. 2007;49(6):753-62.
50. He Y, Liu J, Cai Q, Lv J, Yu F, Chen Q, et al. The pregnancy outcomes in patients with stage 3-4 chronic kidney disease and the effects of pregnancy in the long-term kidney function. J Nephrol. 2018;31(6):953-60.
51. Packham DK, North RA, Fairley KF, Kloss M, Whitworth JA, Kincaid-Smith P. Primary glomerulonephritis and pregnancy. Q J Med. 1989;71(266):537-53.
52. Jungers P, Houillier P, Forget D, Labrunie M, Skhiri H, Giatras I, et al. Influence of pregnancy on the course of primary chronic glomerulonephritis. Lancet. 1995;346(8983):1122-4.
53. Wiles K, Webster P, Seed PT, Bennett-Richards K, Bramham K, Brunskill N, et al. The impact of chronic kidney disease stages 3-5 on pregnancy outcomes. Nephrol Dial Transplant. 2021;36(11):2008-17.
54. Von Hofe J, Bates GW. Ovulation induction. Obstet Gynecol Clin North Am. 2015;42(1):27-37.
55. Martin-Malo A, Benito P, Castillo D, Espinosa M, Burdiel LG, Perez R, et al. Effect of clomiphene citrate on hormonal profile in male hemodialysis and kidney transplant patients. Nephron. 1993;63(4):390-4.
56. Guay AT, Jacobson J, Perez JB, Hodge MB, Velasquez E. Clomiphene increases free testosterone levels in men with both secondary hypogonadism and erectile dysfunction: who does and does not benefit? Int J Impot Res. 2003;15(3):156-65.
57. Rath S, Sharma R, Tarneja P, Chattopadhyay A, Wadhwa R. Ovarian hyperstimulation syndrome during induction of ovulation for intra uterine insemination. Med J Armed Forces India. 2001;57(3):210-2.
58. Garthwaite H, Stewart J, Wilkes S. Multiple pregnancy rate in patients undergoing treatment with clomifene citrate for WHO group II ovulatory disorders: a systematic review. Hum Fertil (Camb). 2021;25(2):1-10.
59. Fertility Problems: Assessment and Treatment. London: National Institute for Health and Care Excellence; 2017. p. 51.
60. Lazarus B, Wu A, Shin JI, Sang Y, Alexander GC, Secora A, et al. Association of metformin use with risk of lactic acidosis across the range of kidney function: a community-based cohort study. JAMA Intern Med. 2018;178(7):903-10.
61. Kar S. Current evidence supporting "letrozole" for ovulation induction. J Hum Reprod Sci. 2013;6(2):93-8.
62. Birken S, Gawinowicz MA, Maydelman Y, Milgrom Y. Metabolism of gonadotropins: comparisons of the primary structures of the human pituitary and urinary LH beta cores and the chimpanzee CG beta core demonstrate universality of core production. J Endocrinol. 2001;171(1):131-41.
63. Nisula BC, Blithe DL, Akar A, Lefort G, Wehmann RE. Metabolic fate of human choriogonadotropin. J Steroid Biochem. 1989;33(4B):733-7.

64. Soni S, Menon MC, Bhaskaran M, Jhaveri KD, Molmenti E, Muoio V. Elevated human chorionic gonadotropin levels in patients with chronic kidney disease: case series and review of literature. Indian J Nephrol. 2013;23(6):424-7.
65. Lin E, Garmo H, Van Hemelrijck M, Zethelius B, Stattin P, Hagström E, et al. Association of gonadotropin-releasing hormone agonists for prostate cancer with cardiovascular disease risk and hypertension in men with diabetes. JAMA Network Open. 2022;5(8):e2225600.
66. Youssef MAFM, Van der Veen F, Al-Inany HG, Mochtar MH, Griesinger G, Nagi Mohesen M, et al. Gonadotropin-releasing hormone agonist versus HCG for oocyte triggering in antagonist-assisted reproductive technology. Cochrane Database Syst Rev. 2014;(10):CD008046.
67. Medscape. Cetrotide (cetrorelix) dosing, indications, interactions, adverse effects, and more. [online] Available from: https://reference.medscape.com/drug/cetrotide-cetrorelix-342750. [Last accessed June, 2023].
68. Perkins KM, Boulet SL, Kissin DM, Jamieson DJ. Risk of ectopic pregnancy associated with assisted reproductive technology in the United States, 2001-2011. Obstet Gynecol. 2015;125(1):70-8.
69. Khalaf Y, Elkington N, Anderson H, Taylor A, Braude P. Ovarian hyperstimulation syndrome and its effect on renal function in a renal transplant patient undergoing IVF treatment: case report. Hum Reprod. 2000;15(6):1275-7.
70. Abou Arkoub R, Xiao CW, Claman P, Clark EG. Acute kidney injury due to ovarian hyperstimulation syndrome. Am J Kidney Dis. 2019;73(3):416-20.
71. Holley JL, Bernardini J, Quadri KH, Greenberg A, Laifer SA. Pregnancy outcomes in a prospective matched control study of pregnancy and renal disease. Clin Nephrol. 1996;45(2):77-82.
72. Sitruk-Ware R. Mifepristone and misoprostol sequential regimen side effects, complications and safety. Contraception. 2006;74(1):48-55.
73. UpToDate. Carboprost tromethamine. [online] Available from: https://www.uptodate.com/contents/search?source=RELATED_SEARCH&search=Carboprost%20tromethamine. [Last accessed June, 2023].
74. Norwitz ER, Edusa V, Park JS. Maternal physiology and complications of multiple pregnancy. Semin Perinatol. 2005;29(5):338-48.
75. Singh N, Malhotra N, Mahey R, Saini M, Patel G, Sethi A. Comparing maternal outcomes in spontaneous singleton pregnancies versus in vitro fertilization conception: single-center 10-year cohort study. JBRA Assist Reprod. 2022;26(4):583-8.
76. Heldal K, Lyngdal PT, Johansen TEB, Kahn JA. Acute renal failure following IVF: case report. Hum Reprod. 2005;20(8):2250-2.
77. Ou YC, Kao YL, Lai SL, Kung FT, Huang FJ, Chang SY, et al. Thromboembolism after ovarian stimulation: successful management of a woman with superior sagittal sinus thrombosis after IVF and embryo transfer: case report. Hum Reprod. 2003;18(11):2375-81.
78. Olausson N, Discacciati A, Nyman AI, Lundberg F, Hovatta O, Westerlund E, et al. Incidence of pulmonary and venous thromboembolism in pregnancies after in vitro fertilization with fresh respectively frozen-thawed embryo transfer: nationwide cohort study. J Thromb Haemost. 2020;18(8):1965-73.
79. Wattanakit K, Cushman M. Chronic kidney disease and venous thromboembolism: epidemiology and mechanisms. Curr Opin Pulm Med. 2009;15(5):408-12.

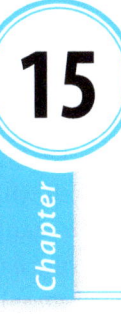

Fertility and Assisted Reproductive Technology in Liver Disorders

Smriti RC Bhatta, Santanu Acharya, Fiona Dennison, Ashis Bassi

■ INTRODUCTION

Liver diseases are on the rise globally. An estimated 1.5 million people, including women in the reproductive age group, had chronic liver diseases in 2017 related to nonalcoholic fatty liver disease (NAFLD), chronic hepatitis B virus (HBV), hepatitis C virus (HCV), autoimmune hepatitis (AIH), and alcohol-related liver disease (ALD).[1] Liver disease impacts fertility and the chances of a successful pregnancy.[2] Consequently, a higher proportion of women are presenting for fertility and pregnancy care, which can be challenging. Knowledge of how chronic liver conditions affect fertility and pregnancy outcomes is useful in providing preconception counseling and appropriately managing them in the fertility and obstetric setting.

This chapter focuses on discussing the fertility implications of chronic liver disease, prepregnancy counseling for these conditions, and specifics for management in the context of assisted reproduction and obstetric care.

■ FERTILITY ISSUES IN CHRONIC LIVER DISEASE

The liver carries out several important endocrine functions, including hormone production, hormone metabolism, and synthesis of sex hormone-binding proteins.[3] Chronic liver dysfunction impacts these functions, and the aspects specifically affecting fertility are altered metabolism of sex hormones and production of sex hormone-binding globulins (SHBG). Altered estrogen metabolism in chronic liver disease can cause oligomenorrhea or amenorrhea, resulting in ovulatory dysfunction. SHBG levels are increased in cirrhosis and result in an alteration of the testosterone-to-estrogen ratio. Low testosterone levels cause decreased libido and testicular atrophy. All of the above create a state of hypogonadotropic hypogonadism affecting both female and male fertility. The impact of the underlying cause of liver disease on fertility is detailed below.

Nonalcoholic fatty liver disease is the most common chronic liver disorder worldwide[4] and is categorized by a buildup of excess fat in the liver, independent of alcohol use. It can be of the nonprogressive type [nonalcoholic fatty liver (NAFL)] or progressive type [nonalcoholic steatohepatitis (NASH)], of which the latter is associated with inflammation and liver damage, leading to cirrhosis. The pathogenesis of NAFLD is complex, and it is linked with metabolic syndrome and insulin resistance. Androgens and estrogens, through their receptors present in the liver, regulate lipid and glucose metabolism, which can therefore be deranged. Men are more commonly affected by NAFLD,[5] and they have a higher prevalence of sexual problems such as erectile dysfunction and hypogonadism.[6] Although premenopausal women are less affected compared to men, those with polycystic ovary syndrome (PCOS) have four times the higher risk of developing NAFLD.[7] The association of NAFLD with metabolic syndrome, obesity, and insulin resistance contributes to endocrine dysfunction, leading to ovulation dysfunction and infertility.

In cases of women with alcoholic liver disease, estrogen metabolism is deranged and causes menstrual cycle irregularity and ovulation problems. Heavy alcohol use may reduce ovarian reserve[8] and increase the incidence of infertility in females.[9] Male fertility is negatively impacted by an effect on reproductive hormone regulation, semen quality, and genetic and epigenetic regulations, resulting in a reduced level of gonadotropins, testosterone, sperm production, and sperm function.[10]

Viral hepatitis is caused by hepatitis A, B, C, D, and E viruses, of which hepatitis B, C, and D (coexist with hepatitis B) have the potential to cause chronic liver disease. Hepatitis B infection is thought to increase the probability of pelvic infection in a female partner through impaired immune response to sexually transmitted infections, resulting in tubal factor infertility.[11] In men with chronic hepatitis B, the virus is present in the semen. Increasing concentrations of viral surface protein cause changes in sperm parameters, increase sperm deoxyribonucleic acid (DNA) damage, and reduce the sperm fertilizing capacity.[12] Similarly, hepatitis C viral infection has a negative impact on sperm parameters.[13] Women of reproductive age with hepatitis C infection experience fertility issues related to reduced ovarian reserve and have fewer live births.[14]

Fertility rates are similar in patients with compensated cirrhosis and the general population, but they are 40% lower in women with a history of decompensation,[15] which may be protective against the increased risks posed by pregnancy in such patients. Women with hepatic cirrhosis display a state of hypothalamic–pituitary–gonadal axis suppression, and a similar effect is seen in men related to high estrogen levels of portal hypertension.[16] Decreased testosterone levels are apparent due to testicular dysfunction, and the degree of dysfunction is linked to the severity of liver disease.[16]

Women with chronic liver diseases contemplating pregnancy should be referred for prepregnancy counseling, and multidisciplinary management is needed in most cases.

■ PREPREGNANCY COUNSELING

Preconception optimization of the underlying liver condition, along with educating women about the implications of pregnancy, is the key to minimizing the risks and promoting a better pregnancy outcome. Counseling is helpful for risk stratification, discussing options to optimize the condition in the nonpregnant state, directing patients to useful resources and support systems, and occasionally discouraging pregnancy if required.

See **Table 1** for general and specific advice related to the condition.[17,18]

TABLE 1: Prepregnancy counseling: General and condition-specific.

Topic/condition	Advice
General advice	• *Contraception:* Enquire about sexual activity and fertility plans. Suggest long-acting reversible contraception (LARC) or other methods combined with barrier contraception to avoid unplanned pregnancy. Use of emergency contraception in all forms is suitable if required • *Medication safety:* Avoid estrogen-containing medications in uncontrolled liver disease and discuss risks related to medications metabolized through the liver for pregnancy and lactation. Consider current treatment methods and safety in pregnancy • *Imaging:* MRI and USS are investigations of choice • Multidisciplinary care involving fertility specialists, obstetricians, hepatologists, and psychosocial support teams
NAFLD	• Lifestyle modification through diet, exercise, and weight loss • *Optimize metabolic comorbidities:* Diabetes, dyslipidemia, and cardiovascular disease
Alcoholic liver disease	• Discuss the risks of fetal alcohol syndrome and delay pregnancy until abstinence is achieved • Decision regarding the use of medications to treat alcohol disorders individualized, based on risk-versus-benefit scenario
Viral hepatitis	• Partners of HBsAg-positive patients should be vaccinated against HBV and use barrier contraception until the viral load of the affected partner is low • HCV patients should be vaccinated for HAV and HBV • Patients with detectable HCV RNA should be treated prior to conceiving • Tenofovir medication of choice in hepatitis B patients • Ribavirin is contraindicated for hepatitis C treatment in pregnancy
Cirrhosis	• Screening for esophageal varices is recommended prepregnancy, and banding is recommended prior to conception. If banding is not feasible, then commence beta-blocker • If the condition deteriorates in pregnancy, an endoscopy can be performed in the second trimester

Contd...

Contd...

Topic/condition	Advice
Autoimmune hepatitis	• Delay pregnancy until a period of disease quiescence to optimize outcomes • Safe to continue steroid treatment and azathioprine during conception and throughout pregnancy
Liver transplant	• Delay the pregnancy for at least 1 year post-transplant with ≥6 months of stable graft function • Calcineurin inhibitors (tacrolimus, cyclosporine), azathioprine, and steroids use is acceptable for pregnancy and lactation, but mycophenolic acid products and mTOR inhibitors are contraindicated

(HAV: hepatitis A virus; HBsAg: hepatitis B surface antigen; HBV: hepatitis B virus; HCV: hepatitis C virus; RNA: ribonucleic acid; MRI: magnetic resonance imaging; mTOR: mammalian target of rapamycin; NAFLD: nonalcoholic fatty liver disease; USS: ultrasound scan)

■ LIVER DISEASE AND ASSISTED REPRODUCTION

Chronic liver disease causes delay in conception due to reasons discussed in the section of fertility issues in chronic liver diseases and couples may require assisted conception. It is important to counsel these women about the process, safety, and success of treatment to help them make an informed decision.[19]

Safety Concerns in Assisted Reproduction

Women requiring fertility treatment are at an increased risk of estrogen-induced deterioration of the liver condition, and biochemical tests are deranged. A case series of 42 women with chronic liver disease (related to viral and AIH), who had undergone 57 cycles of in vitro fertilization (IVF), showed an increased risk of ovarian hyperstimulation syndrome (OHSS), obstetric cholestasis, and preterm birth.[20]

Hepatitis B and C viruses can be transmitted to the embryo through gametes. HBV replication is seen in 40% of female carriers during IVF/intracytoplasmic sperm injection (ICSI) treatment, with the virus detectable in follicular fluid, oocytes, and sperm, potentially posing a risk for transmission to the embryo.[21] HBV and HCV can survive direct exposure to liquid nitrogen and under certain conditions result in cross infection. The steps recommended to minimize risk, prevent vertical transmission, and improve laboratory safety are listed in **Table 2**.

Effect on Assisted Reproduction Treatment

Liver dysfunction can alter the metabolism of gonadotropins used for fertility treatment, resulting in abnormal responses to ovarian stimulation and affecting endometrial receptivity.

TABLE 2: Safety considerations for in vitro fertilization (IVF).[22,23]

IVF steps	Precautions to minimize risk
Pretreatment	Viral load monitoring and required management to achieve a low or undetectable viral load
Oocyte retrieval	Universal precautions when handling blood and body fluids for all patients
Gamete preparation	• Use of sperm "washing" techniques to decrease the viral load • In cases with detectable viral load, process ejaculate in separate centrifuge and hood to prevent cross contamination • Employ cleaning and disinfection procedures between samples
Gamete and embryo cryopreservation	• Specimens with an unknown hepatitis status are individually stored in separate quarantine tanks until the results of infectious disease testing are known • Separate storage tanks for hepatitis B and C-infected patients to protect cryopreserved gametes/embryos from potential cross infection • "Double bagging" or sealing technique to prevent direct contact of cryogenic containers with liquid nitrogen • Sealing straws and vials to limit the potential for leakage of viral agents into their liquid nitrogen storage tanks • Storage of samples in the nitrogen vapor state instead of the liquid phase

The number of oocytes retrieved and IVF success rates are decreased even with moderate alcohol use in cases with alcoholic liver disease.[24]

Effect on Assisted Reproduction Treatment Outcome

Hepatitis B infection does not impact the outcome of IVF/ICSI treatment.[25] Based on a study that included data from 25 retrospective cohort studies involving more than 19,269 couples, there was no reduction in the clinical pregnancy or live birth rate seen in cases where both partners were affected by hepatitis B.[26]

In cases of NAFLD, the presence of comorbidities such as high body mass index (BMI) and type 2 diabetes is associated with lower live birth rates in women with IVF.

■ OBSTETRIC CONCERNS

Pregnancy in a patient with established liver disease is considered high risk due to increased maternal and fetal complications. Pregnancy affects the liver physiology, and liver disorders affect the pregnancy outcome.

Changes to Liver Physiology in Pregnancy

Pregnancy influences liver functions, as depicted in **Figures 1 and 2**. Most changes normalize within 2 weeks of delivery but can take up to 12 weeks.

Obstetric Concerns Specific to the Condition

Nonalcoholic Fatty Liver Disease

Nonalcoholic fatty liver disease is the most common cause of cirrhosis in pregnancy[27] and can lead to adverse maternal and fetal outcomes, including miscarriages,[28] hypertensive disease, gestational diabetes, postpartum hemorrhage, and preterm birth.[29] The prevalence of NAFLD in pregnancy has tripled over the last decade.[29]

A recent study on women with NAFLD from a South Asian population showed a twofold higher risk of gestational hypertension and preeclampsia in pregnancy compared to non-NAFLD cases after adjusting for confounding

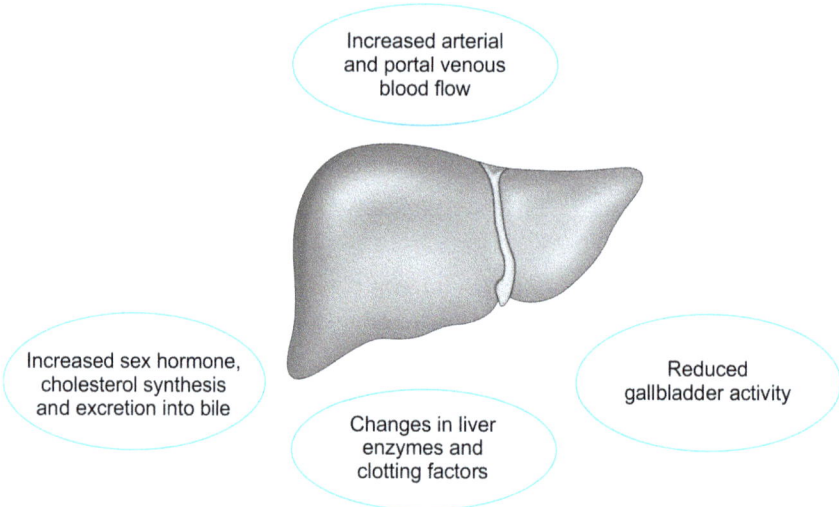

Fig. 1: Liver: physiological changes in pregnancy.

Increased ↑	Decreased ↓	No change ↔
• Total cholesterol, triglyceride, fibrinogen, and ceruloplasmin • ALP and AFP • Factors I, II, V, VI, VIII, X, XII, and fibrinogen and ceruloplasmin	• Albumin • AT 3, proteins C and S • Occasional—GGT and bilirubin	• AST, ALT, and PT • Platelet

Fig. 2: Liver function and hematological changes in pregnancy. (AFP: alpha-fetoprotein; ALP: alkaline phosphatase; ALT: alanine aminotransferase; AST: aspartate aminotransferase; GGT: gamma-glutamyltransferase; PT: prothrombin time)

factors.[30] Another Swedish study,[31] which analyzed 110 births with maternal NAFLD, between 1992 and 2001, found that women with NAFLD had a higher risk of gestational diabetes mellitus (GDM) [adjusted relative risk (aRR) 2.78; 95% confidence interval (CI) 1.25–6.15], preeclampsia (aRR 1.95; 95% CI 1.03–3.70), cesarean section (aRR 1.52; 95% CI 1.19–1.94), low birth weight (aRR 2.40; 95% CI 1.21–4.78), and very preterm (<32 weeks) delivery (aRR 6.92; 95% CI 2.96–16.14). NAFLD independently increased the risk of preeclampsia and GDM in women with BMI <30 kg/m^2.

Hepatitis

The five hepatitis viruses affecting the liver have variable modes of transmission, course, and impact on pregnancy, which are detailed in **Table 3**.[32,33] Mandatory screening for hepatitis B, hepatitis C, and human immunodeficiency virus (HIV) infections is recommended to all couples proceeding with assisted reproduction, with a view to risk reduction in pregnancy by reducing viral load in the affected partner/s and immunizing the nonaffected partner.

Autoimmune Hepatitis

Autoimmune hepatitis is a multifactorial progressive liver disease that predominantly affects women in their childbearing years but can occur at any age. The incidence in the general population is 1:100,000, and it can lead to liver cirrhosis.[34] Pregnancy can cause deterioration of the condition, and treatment should be optimized prior to considering conception. Studies have shown that 20% of women can have a flare during pregnancy although more likely in the postpartum period.[35] There is an increase in miscarriage, fetal growth restriction, and preterm birth. Treatment is often a combination of azathioprine and prednisolone. Both of these can be continued during pregnancy if felt that the benefits outweigh the risks. Women on long-term steroids will require screening for gestational diabetes and increased steroid coverage for delivery.

Hepatic Hemangioma

Hepatic hemangiomas are the most common benign liver tumors and are most frequently diagnosed in women of reproductive age (age 30–50 years). Hemangiomas are asymptomatic and usually an incidental finding detected on ultrasound imaging, either prior to or occasionally during pregnancy. These are frequently small in size (<4 cm), but can grow in pregnancy due to the physiological changes and stimulation from increased estrogen levels.

An abdominal ultrasound scan at the start of pregnancy can provide a baseline measurement to assess whether the hemangioma is increasing in size. A growing lesion may present with right upper quadrant pain, nausea, or,

TABLE 3: Hepatitis viruses: Transmission and risks in pregnancy.

Hepatitis type	Mode of transmission	Course	Maternal-to-child transmission	Maternal risks	Fetal risks
Hepatitis A	Fecal–oral	Acute, self-limiting	Rare but reported	Preterm labor, placental abruption, and premature rupture of membranes	Fetal liver injury
Hepatitis B	Sexual and contact with infected body fluids	Acute, potential to become chronic	Vertical transmission, transplacental transmission if breaks in maternal–fetal barrier with invasive procedures such as CVS, amniocentesis, FBS, and application of fetal scalp electrode	Gestational diabetes, miscarriage and preterm delivery, worsening of liver disease, and progression to cirrhosis	Prematurity
Hepatitis C	Infected blood and other body fluids, sexual contact	Acute, potential to become chronic	• Vertical transmission, 5% with viremia and 10% with HIV coinfection • Increase risk with invasive procedures such as CVS, amniocentesis, FBS, and application of fetal scalp electrode	• Gestational diabetes, APH, PPH, and preterm labor • 20-fold increased risk of obstetric cholestasis • Worsening of liver disease	Prematurity, small-for-gestational-age, low birth weight, and intrauterine fetal death
Hepatitis D	Infected blood and blood products	Coinfection with hepatitis B	Vertical transmission rare	Same as hepatitis B	Same as hepatitis B
Hepatitis E	Fecal–oral route	Acute, mild, and self-limiting	Vertical transmission	Miscarriage, fulminant hepatitis, preterm birth, and stillbirth	Prematurity and low birth weight

(APH: antepartum hemorrhage; CVS: chorionic villus sampling; FBS: fetal blood sampling; HIV: human immunodeficiency virus; PPH: postpartum hemorrhage) more likely, no change to symptoms. If the hemangioma is increasing in size, there is a risk of rupture during pregnancy. The patient may present with acute abdominal pain, shock, collapse, and fetal distress, which can be difficult to distinguish from placental abruption in the acute setting. Liver function tests will remain normal throughout, but serial imaging during pregnancy can detect growing lesions.

Alcoholic Liver Disease

Alcohol-related liver disease and alcohol consumption during pregnancy are linked to adverse pregnancy outcomes. The safe level of alcohol consumption during pregnancy is not known, and therefore the safest approach advised is to avoid alcohol altogether to minimize risks.[36]

A study[37] on 2,440 women with alcoholic liver disease before and after delivery found that there was an increased risk of moderate and very preterm birth [adjusted odds ratio (OR) 1.53; 95% CI 1.37–1.72 and 1.15–2.06, respectively], small-for-gestational-age infants (adjusted OR 1.22; 95% CI 1.05–1.43), and low Apgar scores (<7) at 5 minutes (adjusted OR 1.49; 95% CI 1.15–1.92). All the risks were found to be higher in those admitted to the hospital with known liver disease pre delivery.

Cirrhosis

Preexisting liver disease due to any etiology can worsen during pregnancy, leading to cirrhosis, and some women enter pregnancy with a diagnosis of cirrhosis. For patients with cirrhosis, the degree of hepatic decompensation is important when considering assisted reproduction, with caution used in those with advanced or decompensated cirrhosis. There is no absolute contraindication to assisted reproduction in women with cirrhosis or prior transplant.[17] Preconception counseling for risk stratification is recommended.

The pregnancy course of cases with cirrhosis is influenced by the severity of the liver disease. The Child–Turcotte–Pugh calculator estimates the cirrhosis severity, and higher scores predict worse pregnancy outcomes.[38] Another predictor for outcome in cirrhotic pregnant women is the model for end-stage liver disease score (MELD score), where women with a MELD score of <6 have minimal complications and those with a score of >10 predict hepatic decompensation in pregnancy.[39] Worsening and decompensation lead to complications of ascites, hepatic encephalopathy, coagulopathy, splenic artery aneurysmal rupture, and portal hypertension.[40] Pregnancy is therefore high risk, with increased maternal and fetal morbidity and rarely mortality. Furthermore, diuretics and spironolactone are contraindicated in pregnancy, and stopping at conception is recommended.

A national population-based cohort study[41] identified 103 cases of women with cirrhosis from a cohort of 1.3 million women and found that these pregnancies were at an increased risk of cesarean delivery (36 vs. 16%, respectively; aRR 2.00; 95% CI 1.47–2.73), low birth weight (15 vs. 3%; aRR 3.87; 95% CI 2.11–7.06), and preterm delivery (19 vs. 5%; aRR 3.51; 95% CI 2.16–5.72). The risk of gestational diabetes, preeclampsia, small-for-gestational-age, congenital malformations, stillbirth, and maternal mortality was not increased.

Another US population-based study[42] reported that pregnancies with cirrhosis more than doubled over the past decade. An increased risk of adverse events including hypertensive disease, postpartum hemorrhage, and preterm birth was noted. However, the maternal mortality rate was rare (≤1%).

Besides maternal and fetal outcomes, postpartum liver complications in women with cirrhosis were investigated in a Canadian study.[15] Findings showed that <2% of women had liver-related complications, and these were significantly higher in decompensated (13%) than in compensated cirrhosis (1.2%) ($p < 0.001$).

The most recent systematic review and meta-analysis[43] included 11 studies, comprising 2,912 pregnancies in women with cirrhosis, from 1982 to 2020 of which seven studies were eligible for inclusion in the meta-analysis. The study found an overall mortality rate to be 0.89% with 70% of cases linked to variceal bleeding during vaginal delivery. There was a higher chance of preterm delivery (OR 6.7; 95% CI 5.1–9.1), cesarean section (OR 2.6; 95% CI 1.7–3.9), preeclampsia (OR 3.8; 95% CI 2.2–6.5), and small-for-gestational-age neonates (OR 2.6; 95% CI 1.6–4.2) compared to the general obstetric population.

Pregnancies with cirrhosis, although rare, can be challenging, and multidisciplinary management is essential to improve outcomes and reduce maternal mortality.

Portal Hypertension

Portal hypertension is a consequence of chronic liver disease and increases mortality risk. Increased pressure in the portal vein can be due to a blockage or increased resistance from the cirrhotic liver. This, combined with increased cardiac output in pregnancy and pressure of the gravid uterus on the inferior vena cava, increases the portal system blood flow which is rerouted and causes varices, most commonly in the esophagus. Variceal bleeding presents acutely and needs emergency management with medications or surgery in the form of endoscopic band ligation or portocaval shunt surgery.

Pregnancy is a high-risk situation due to the physiological hemodynamic changes in pregnancy. A recent review[44] included information from 26 studies and presented information on 891 pregnancies from 581 patients with portal hypertension. Results showed that 10% of patients developed portal hypertension in pregnancy, and there was higher mortality related to complications of variceal bleeding and hepatic decompensation. The most common complication was thrombocytopenia (41%, 95% CI 23-60%), and there was an increased risk of miscarriages (14%, 95% CI 8-20%), preterm birth (27%, 95% CI 19-37%), low birth weights (22%, 95% CI 15-30%), and postpartum hemorrhage [relative risk (RR) 5.09; 95% CI 1.84-14.12]. A beta-blocker should be commenced in pregnancy, if not already instigated, and should continue throughout.

The optimal mode of delivery is controversial as there is a risk of bleeding for variceal rupture during vaginal delivery, and cesarean section may increase the risk of hemorrhage due to portal hypertensive collaterals. The mode of delivery, therefore, should be guided by obstetric indication.[17]

Liver Transplant

Liver transplant in cirrhosis patients can improve the chances of conception.[45] For liver transplant recipients, the stability of graft function should be assessed when considering assisted reproduction.

Pregnancy outcomes after liver transplant are favorable, but the risk of maternal and fetal complications is increased.[46] Adverse outcomes include placental abruption, coagulopathy, hypertension, operative birth, and postpartum hemorrhage.[47]

In the first year post-transplant, there is an increased risk of infection and graft rejection. Therefore, women are advised to delay pregnancy for at least a year post-transplant.

Frequent monitoring of graft function is recommended during pregnancy and in the postpartum period. Tacrolimus is the immunosuppressive of choice in pregnancy, and levels should be monitored every 2-4 weeks. Dosage should be guided by levels and liver tests. Breastfeeding in women receiving tacrolimus has not shown any adverse events.

■ CONCLUSION

Chronic liver diseases due to various underlying etiologies are rising globally and affect women of reproductive age. Liver dysfunction reduces fertility due to its impact on the hormone production and metabolic functions of the liver, creating a state of hypogonadotropic hypogonadism affecting both female and male fertility. Preconception counseling and optimal management of the underlying condition are recommended to minimize risk and improve the safety of assisted conception and its outcomes. Pregnancy in women with chronic liver diseases is at high risk with increased maternal and fetal adverse events. Close monitoring, timely intervention, and multidisciplinary management are required to enhance the chances of a successful pregnancy.

KEY LEARNING POINTS

- To understand the fertility issues in chronic liver disease.
- To be aware of the general and condition specific prepregnancy counseling requirements.
- To understand the implications of chronic liver disease in assisted reproduction.
- To have knowledge of general changes in the liver physiology in pregnancy and obstetric concerns related to specific liver conditions.

■ REFERENCES

1. GBD 2017 Disease and Injury Incidence and Prevalence Collaborators. Global, regional, and national incidence, prevalence, and years lived with disability for 354 diseases and injuries for 195 countries and territories, 1990-2017: a systematic analysis for the Global Burden of Disease Study 2017. Lancet 2018;392:1789-858.
2. Golabi P, Fazel S, Otgonsuren M, Escheik C, Sayiner M, Younossi ZM. Association of parity in patients with chronic liver disease. Ann Hepatol. 2018;17(6):1035-41.
3. Rhyu J, Yu R. Newly discovered endocrine functions of the liver. World J Hepatol. 2021;13(11):1611-28.
4. Sayiner M, Koenig A, Henry L, Younossi ZM. Epidemiology of nonalcoholic fatty liver disease and nonalcoholic steatohepatitis in the United States and the rest of the world. Clin Liver Dis. 2016;20:205-14.
5. Ballestri S, Nascimbeni F, Baldelli E, Marrazzo A, Romagnoli D, Lonardo A. NAFLD as a sexual dimorphic disease: role of gender and reproductive status in the development and progression of nonalcoholic fatty liver disease and inherent cardiovascular risk. Adv Ther. 2017;34:1291-326.
6. Hawksworth DJ, Burnett AL. Nonalcoholic fatty liver disease, male sexual dysfunction, and infertility: common links, common problems. Sex Med Rev. 2020;8(2):274-85.
7. Asfari MM, Sarmini MT, Baidoun F, Al-Khadra Y, Ezzaizi Y, Dasarathy S, et al. Association of non-alcoholic fatty liver disease and polycystic ovarian syndrome. BMJ Open Gastroenterol. 2020;7:e000352.
8. Hawkins Bressler L, Bernardi LA, De Chavez PJD, Baird DD, Carnethon MR, Marsh EE. Alcohol, cigarette smoking, and ovarian reserve in reproductive-age African-American women. Am J Obstet Gynecol. 2016;215:758.e1-e9.
9. Tolstrup JS, Kjaer S, Holst C, Sharif H, Munk C, Osler M, et al. Alcohol use as predictor for infertility in a representative population of Danish women. Acta Obs Gynecol Scand. 2003;82:744-9.
10. Finelli R, Mottola F, Agarwal A. Impact of alcohol consumption on male fertility potential: a narrative review. Int J Environ Res Public Health. 2022;19(1):328.
11. Lao TT, Mak JSM, Li TC. Hepatitis B virus infection status and infertility causes in couples seeking fertility treatment—indicator of impaired immune response? Am J Reprod Immunol. 2017;77(4):e12636.
12. Han TT, Huang JH, Gu J, Xie QD, Zhong Y, Huang TH. Hepatitis B virus surface protein induces sperm dysfunction through the activation of a Bcl2/Bax signaling cascade triggering AIF/Endo G-mediated apoptosis. Andrology. 2021;9(3):944-55.

13. Karamolahi S, Yazdi RS, Zangeneh M, Makiani MJ, Farhoodi B, Gilani MAS. Impact of hepatitis B virus and hepatitis C virus infection on sperm parameters of infertile men. Int J Reprod Biomed. 2019;17(8):551-6.
14. Karampatou A, Han X, Kondili LA, Taliani G, Ciancio A, Morisco F, et al. Premature ovarian senescence and a high miscarriage rate impair fertility in women with HCV. J Hepatol. 2017;68(1):33-41.
15. Flemming JA, Mullin M, Lu J, Sarkar MA, Djerboua M, Velez MP, et al. Outcomes of pregnant women with cirrhosis and their infants in a population-based study. Gastroenterology. 2020;159(5):1752-62.e10.
16. Neong SF, Billington EO, Congly SE. Sexual dysfunction and sex hormone abnormalities in patients with cirrhosis: review of pathogenesis and management. Hepatology. 2019;69:2683-95.
17. Sarkar M, Brady CW, Fleckenstein J, Forde KA, Khungar V, Molleston JP, et al. Reproductive health and liver disease: practice guidance by the American Association for the Study of Liver Diseases. Hepatology. 2021;73(1):318-65.
18. Arora A, Kumar A, Anand AC, Puri P, Dhiman RK, Acharya SK, et al. Indian National Association for the Study of the Liver-Federation of Obstetric and Gynaecological Societies of India Position Statement on management of liver diseases in pregnancy. J Clin Exp Hepatol. 2019;9(3):383-406.
19. Flemming JA, Velez MP. The ART of medicine: counselling women with liver disease about assisted reproductive technology. J Hepatol. 2021;74(6):1283-5.
20. Rahim MN, Theocharidou E, Yen Lau KG, Ahmed R, Marattukalam F, Long L, et al. Safety and efficacy of in vitro fertilisation in patients with chronic liver disease and liver transplantation recipients. J Hepatol. 2021;74(6):1407-15.
21. Mak JSM, Lao TT, Leung MBW, Chung CHS, Chung JPW, Cheung LP, et al. Ovarian HBV replication following ovulation induction in female hepatitis B carriers undergoing IVF treatment: a prospective observational study. J Viral Hepat. 2020;27(2):110-7.
22. Practice Committee of the American Society for Reproductive Medicine. Recommendations for reducing the risk of viral transmission during fertility treatment with the use of autologous gametes: a committee opinion. Fertil Steril. 2020;114(6):1158-64.
23. Shapiro H, Zaman L, Kennedy VL, Dean N, Yudin MH, Loutfy M. Managing and preventing blood-borne viral infection transmission in assisted reproduction: a Canadian Fertility and Andrology Society clinical practice guideline. Reprod Biomed Online. 2020;41(2):203-16.
24. Van Heertum K, Rossi B. Alcohol and fertility: how much is too much? Fertil Res Pract. 2017;3:10.
25. Mak JSM, Lao TT. Assisted reproduction in hepatitis carrier couples. Best Pract Res Clin Obstet Gynaecol. 2020;68:103-8.
26. Xiong Y, Liu C, Wei W, Huang S, Wang J, Qi Y, et al. The impact of biparental hepatitis B virus infection on pregnancy outcomes in patients undergoing assisted reproductive technology treatment: a systematic review and meta-analysis. Arch Gynecol Obstet. 2022;306:1253-66.
27. Sarkar M, Djerboua M, Flemming JA. NAFLD cirrhosis is rising among childbearing women and is the most common cause of cirrhosis in pregnancy. Clin Gastroenterol Hepatol. 2022;20(2):e315-8.

28. Koralegedara IS, Warnasekara JN, Dayaratne KG, De Silva FN, Premadasa JK, Agampodi SB. Non-alcoholic fatty liver disease (NAFLD): a significant predictor of gestational diabetes mellitus (GDM) and early pregnancy miscarriages—prospective study in Rajarata Pregnancy Cohort (RaPCo). BMJ Open Gastroenterol. 2022;9:e000831.
29. Sarkar M, Grab J, Dodge JL, Gunderson EP, Rubin J, Irani RA, et al. Non-alcoholic fatty liver disease in pregnancy is associated with adverse maternal and perinatal outcomes. J Hepatol. 2020;73:516-22.
30. Abeysekara V, Kodithuwakku SUA, Herath HP. Non-alcoholic fatty liver disease and pregnancy complications among Sri Lankan women: a cross-sectional analytical study. PLoS One. 2019;14(4):e0215326.
31. Hagström H, Höijer J, Ludvigsson JF, Bottai M, Ekbom A, Hultcrantz R, et al. Adverse outcomes of pregnancy in women with non-alcoholic fatty liver disease. Liver Int. 2016;36(2):268-74.
32. Terrault NA, Levy MT, Cheung KW, Jourdain G. Viral hepatitis and pregnancy. Nat Rev Gastroenterol Hepatol. 2021;18:117-30.
33. Asafo-Agyei KO, Samant H. Pregnancy and viral hepatitis. In: StatPearls [Internet]. Treasure Island (FL): StatPearls Publishing; 2022.
34. Autoimmune Hepatitis and Pregnancy. [online] Available from: https://www.ncbi.nlm.nih.gov/books/NBK544270/. [Last accessed June, 2023].
35. Peters MG. Management of autoimmune hepatitis in pregnant women. Gastroenterol Hepatol (N Y). 2017;13(8):504-6.
36. Fetal alcohol spectrum disorder. [online] Available from: https://www.nice.org.uk/guidance/qs204/chapter/Quality-statement-1-Advice-on-avoiding-alcohol-in-pregnancy. [Last accessed June, 2023].
37. Stokkeland K, Ebrahim F, Hultcrantz R, Ekbom A, Stephansson O. Mothers with alcoholic liver disease and the risk for preterm and small-for-gestational-age birth. Alcohol Alcohol. 2013;48(2):166-71.
38. Gao X, Zhu Y, Liu H, Yu H, Wang M. Maternal and fetal outcomes of patients with liver cirrhosis: a case-control study. BMC Pregnancy Childbirth. 2021;21:280.
39. Westbrook RH, Yeoman AD, O'Grady JG, Harrison PM, Devlin J, Heneghan MA. Model for end-stage liver disease score predicts outcome in cirrhotic patients during pregnancy. Clin Gastroenterol Hepatol. 2011;9:694-9.
40. Rahim MN, Pirani T, Williamson C, Heneghan MA. Management of pregnancy in women with cirrhosis. United European Gastroenterol J. 2021;9(1):110-9.
41. Hagström H, Höijer J, Marschall HU, Williamson C, Heneghan MA, Westbrook RH, et al. Outcomes of pregnancy in mothers with cirrhosis: a national population-based cohort study of 1.3 million pregnancies. Hepatol Commun. 2018;2:1299-305.
42. Huang AC, Grab J, Flemming JA, Dodge JL, Irani RA, Sarkar M. Pregnancies with cirrhosis are rising and associated with adverse maternal and perinatal outcomes. Am J Gastroenterol. 2022;117(3):445-52.
43. van der Slink LL, Scholten I, van Etten-Jamaludin FS, Takkenberg RB, Painter RC. Pregnancy in women with liver cirrhosis is associated with increased risk for complications: a systematic review and meta-analysis of the literature. BJOG. 2022;129:1644-52.

44. Pal K, Sadanandan DM, Gupta A, Nayak D, Pyakurel M, Keepanasseril A, et al. Maternal and perinatal outcome in pregnancies complicated with portal hypertension: a systematic review and meta-analysis. Hepatol Int. 2023;17(1):170-9.
45. Dokmak A, Trivedi HD, Bonder A, Wolf J. Pregnancy in chronic liver disease: before and after transplantation. Ann Hepatol. 2021;26:100557.
46. Valentin N, Guerrido I, Rozenshteyn F, Pinotti R, Wu YC, Collins K, et al. Pregnancy outcomes after liver transplantation: a systematic review and meta-analysis. Am J Gastroenterol. 2021;116(3):491-504.
47. Thornton AT, Huang Y, Mourad MJ, Wright JD, D'Alton ME, Friedman AM. Obstetric outcomes among women with a liver transplant. J Matern Fetal Neonatal Med. 2021;34(18):2932-7.

16

Fertility and Assisted Reproductive Technology in Hypertensive Disorders

Atri Pal, Sujoy Dasgupta

■ INTRODUCTION

Throughout the world, there is an increased acceptance of infertility treatment and in vitro fertilization (IVF). Women seeking infertility treatment are usually older and they have a greater risk of age-related chronic medical conditions such as hypertension. Chronic hypertension is associated with poor outcomes of pregnancy.[1] It is of concern that in women having chronic metabolic conditions, assisted reproductive technology (ART) may further augment the perinatal risks associated with chronic hypertension such as placental abruption, prematurity, fetal growth restriction, and neonatal mortality.[2]

The risk of placental-mediated complications is higher in mothers with chronic hypertension who conceive through ART as compared to normotensive women who have unassisted pregnancies.[2] This may be due to negative synergistic effects on development and placental implantation. The ovarian stimulation causes a marked increase of plasma renin and also aldosterone excretion in urine in coordination with the increase in plasma and estradiol.[3] The use of these exogenous hormones may affect the renin–angiotensin system, which will lead to high blood pressure by exogenous hormones and aggravate the condition during IVF stimulation.

Hypertension also has a profound effect on male fertility. Though there is a paucity of studies, existing data have demonstrated that hypertensive men are more likely to have semen abnormalities compared to men who are normotensive.[4] Moreover, certain antihypertensives have an adverse effect on sperm quality as well as fertilization capacity.

Due to the synergistic effect of ART and hypertension, it is prudent for the clinician to treat a couple with chronic hypertension, who has come for fertility treatment, systematically from preconception counseling through tailored ART to proper pregnancy care. Our aim should be to keep the patients' blood pressure under control, prevent the occurrence of preeclampsia/eclampsia, and help the couple achieve a live birth of a healthy baby without an increase in morbidity and mortality. In this chapter, we are going to evaluate the management of an infertile couple who is hypertensive and has come for ART treatment.

PRECONCEPTION COUNSELING IN WOMEN WITH HYPERTENSION (BOX 1)

Preconception counseling is of utmost importance for a couple with hypertension coming for infertility treatment. According to guidelines, systolic blood pressure should be maintained under 150 mm Hg and diastolic blood pressure should be under 100 mm Hg, irrespective of whether target organ damage is present or not.[5]

Hypertensive women, who are considering pregnancy, should undergo investigations including serum creatinine level, complete blood count, and hepatic transaminase.[5] Additional testing such as electrocardiogram might be included for detecting left ventricular hypertrophy.[5] In patients who have poorly controlled disease or those who have known kidney or heart disease, other evaluation such as those for hypertensive retinopathy for target organ damage can be considered.[6]

According to data which is largely based on retrospective data, methyldopa (α-adrenergic agonist) and labetalol (a combined α- and β-adrenergic blocking agent) are first-line medications for hypertension during pregnancy. Labetalol is preferred over methyldopa because it is less likely to cause fatigue. Moreover, methyldopa may lead to drug-induced lupus erythematosus. Long-acting formulations of calcium channel blockers such as nifedipine can be used as an additional second-line agent when blood pressure is not controlled adequately by methyldopa or labetalol. Propranolol and atenolol have been associated with premature labor and intrauterine growth restriction, respectively. Therefore, these drugs should

BOX 1: Preconception counseling in women with hypertension.

Check the blood pressure of the woman
- Target blood pressure: 150/100 mm Hg

Check the BMI of the woman
- If the patient is overweight or obese, advise weight reduction

Reassess the medication the patient is receiving, adjust the dose if required, and change the medicine to pregnancy safe antihypertensives
- Pregnancy safe medication:
  - *First line:* Methyldopa and labetalol
  - *Second line:* Nifedipine

Advise investigations to check for end-organ damage and other comorbidities
- *For kidney:* Serum creatinine, spot urine protein-to-creatinine ratio
- *For liver:* Alanine aminotransferase (ALT) and aspartate aminotransferase (AST)
- *For eye:* Check for hypertensive retinopathy
- *For diabetes:* Fasting blood sugar and glycosylated hemoglobin
- *For heart:* ECG, echocardiography

(BMI: body mass index; ECG: electrocardiography)

BOX 2: Antihypertensives to be avoided.

- Angiotensin-converting enzyme (ACE) inhibitors
- Diuretics
- Angiotensin receptor blockers
- Propranolol, atenolol

not be used during pregnancy. Angiotensin receptor blockers (ARBs) and angiotensin-converting enzyme (ACE) inhibitors must be avoided during pregnancy because they are associated with serious fetal anomalies such as cardiovascular malformation, renal dysgenesis, and malformations of the central nervous system **(Box 2)**. Therefore, it is of prime importance that clinicians take cognizance of the patient's medical history and what medicines the patient is taking and change the medicines accordingly.

Studies have demonstrated that maternal prepregnancy body mass index (BMI) is positively associated with the risk of hypertensive disorders of pregnancy (HDP).[7] Visceral obesity and excess weight gain are major causes of hypertension, accounting for nearly 65–75% of the risk for essential hypertension.[8] Therefore, weight reduction must be emphasized by clinicians before starting ART. In a recent systemic review, reduction of sodium intake from an average high sodium intake level to an average intake below the recommended upper level of 5.8 g/day, decrease in mean arterial pressure (MAP) of about 4 mm Hg in patients with hypertension.[9] Keeping this in mind, a woman who is going for ART treatment and trying to conceive must be advised and encouraged to maintain low dietary sodium intake.

Dyslipidemia influences the risk of hypertension significantly.[10] It is not uncommon that patients with hypertension have associated dyslipidemia and are on medications such as statins to treat this condition. Statins have been traditionally categorized as Category "X" drug. Therefore, women who are receiving statins should be properly counseled and their drugs should be modified into pregnancy-safe medications.

Moreover, other comorbidities which are frequently associated with chronic hypertension, such as obesity and diabetes mellitus, must be screened properly and, if present, duly optimized before IVF.

Usually, kidneys are the first end-organ that are affected by chronic hypertension. Baseline renal function assessment is of prime importance. This includes serum creatinine, spot urine protein-to-creatinine ratio, and 24-hour urinary collection for total protein clearance. Spot urine protein-to-creatinine ratio <0.15 indicates proteinuria <300 mg for a 24-hour sample and, in the absence of abnormal serum creatinine, usually does not warrant evaluation with 24-hour urine collection.

Antihypertensive medications also have a profound effect on male fertility. Studies have demonstrated that Ca^{2+} channel blockers cause inhibition of acrosomal exocytosis.[11] Intake of calcium antagonists for control of hypertension may lead to reversible male infertility which can be associated with IVF failure.[11] Various other studies have associated calcium channel blockers with reduced fertilization capacity of sperm. It is important to evaluate the husband's medical history and change the medicine from calcium channel blockers to safer medicines such as ACE inhibitors and ARBs.

Multidisciplinary team care is an important cornerstone for patients with chronic hypertension during preconception counseling and antepartum and postpartum periods. A cardiologist's opinion has to be taken for optimizing the medication and titrating the dose to maintain the blood pressure within desired levels. If kidney function test is abnormal, a nephrologist's opinion has to be taken. An ophthalmologist's opinion must be taken to rule out retinopathy. A dietician's advice for adequate weight control is desirable.

Realistic counseling regarding the risk of development of preeclampsia (which is reported to be around 22%), eclampsia, and hemolysis, elevated liver enzymes, and low platelets (HELLP) syndrome in case of chronic hypertensive women undergoing IVF is recommended. The antenatal risks including placental abruption, postpartum hemorrhage, renal insufficiency, myocardial infarction, stroke, preterm delivery, intrauterine fetal demise (IUFD), and fetal growth restriction must be discussed. The increased risk of cesarean section, admission to intensive care unit (ICU), and maternal morbidity and mortality must also be explained to the patient with clarity.

Thus, before moving onto ART, a couple where either partner has hypertension must receive a pragmatic preconception counseling which must encompass dietary and lifestyle modification, weight reduction, and modification of the ongoing medication.

ASSISTED REPRODUCTIVE TECHNOLOGY IN WOMEN WITH HYPERTENSION

As has been discussed before, the use of these exogenous hormones may affect the renin–angiotensin system which will lead to high blood pressure by exogenous hormones and aggravate the condition during IVF stimulation. Therefore, our aim should be to decrease the dose of gonadotropin injections, and patient-tailored, personalized IVF treatment should be done.

Ovarian stimulation is an integral part of IVF. The aim of ovarian stimulation is to obtain the optimum number of oocytes so that the couple has the best probability of having a live birth. Though an increase of gonadotropin dose usually yields a higher number of oocytes,[12] this is also associated with an increased risk of ovarian hyperstimulation syndrome (OHSS) and increase of serum estradiol. One case–control study has indicated that ART [IVF/intracytoplasmic sperm injection (ICSI)]-mediated pregnancies, which were complicated with severe OHSS, may be related to gestational hypertension.[13] To mitigate the problem of pregnancy complicated by OHSS, elective cryopreservation of embryos and frozen embryo transfer (FET) have been advocated. However, FET itself has been associated with an increased risk of gestational hypertension.[14,15] In ovulatory women with infertility and also in elderly poor ovarian responders, there is no significant difference in live birth rate between FET and fresh embryo transfer.[16,17] Therefore, fresh embryo transfer can be planned provided the number of oocytes retrieved is less and the risk of OHSS is low. Using a low dose of gonadotropins (minimum stimulation) can be another possible way to mitigate the problem.

Letrozole has often been used in combination with gonadotropins for controlled ovarian hyperstimulation (COH) during IVF. It inhibits the aromatase enzyme and thereby reduces the serum estradiol level in the body. It has been reported by studies that the supraphysiological serum estrogen level that is attained during IVF treatment is suppressed with letrozole cotreatment to a more physiological level.[18] Studies have shown that cotreatment with letrozole during COH improves the outcome of IVF in normal responders. It helps in increasing the number of blastocysts obtained; moreover, it does not increase the risk of OHSS.[19] It has also been demonstrated by various studies that the use of concomitant letrozole during COH decreases the consumption of exogenous follicle-stimulating hormone (FSH) during the stimulation.[20] Therefore, by decreasing the estradiol level and dose of gonadotropin, letrozole may be beneficial and protective in patients with hypertension. However, it must also be noted that there are no direct studies evaluating the effect of letrozole on chronic hypertension during IVF stimulation and fresh transfer cycle.

Although FET decreases the risk of OHSS even in normoresponders, it has traditionally been associated with an increased risk of HDP. However, with the advancement in the field of infertility, newer protocols for FET have been introduced, which may help us mitigate the problem of HDP after FET. It has been postulated that in programmed FET, there is ineffective decidualization which leads to impaired placental function.[21] Moreover, it has been suggested by recent studies that due to the absence of corpus luteum and thereby relaxin, which is produced by corpus luteum during pregnancy, there is an increased risk of hypertensive disorders in pregnancies conceived after programmed FET.[22] Recent studies have demonstrated that natural cycle FET and stimulated cycle FET can help mitigate this problem. Saito et al., using Japanese Assisted Reproductive Technology Registry data, compared outcomes in over 100,000 patients undergoing hormone replacement cycle or natural cycle FET. They reported that the pregnancies conceived in a hormone replacement cycle FET had increased the risk of HDP.[23] Similar conclusions have been derived from other studies.[24,25] In recent years, there has been an increased trend of stimulated cycle FET. In this, oral ovulogens and/or injectable gonadotropins are used to induce ovulation and FET is performed in that cycle after ovulation. Studies have confirmed that pregnancies conceived after stimulated cycle FET have a lower risk of HDP. Moreover, in stimulated cycles (with letrozole), the endometrial thickness is significantly more than that of hormone replacement FET. It has been reported that thin endometrium during embryo transfer is associated with an increased risk of pregnancy-induced hypertension. Though data regarding the outcome of type of FET cycle on chronic hypertension is lacking, it is prudent enough to advise hypertensive women to undergo a natural cycle or stimulated cycle FET.

Twin pregnancies are associated with an increased risk of hypertensive disorders in pregnancies.[26] Therefore, in patients who are already hypertensive, a pragmatic approach would be to decrease the risk of twin or multifetal gestation. Single embryo transfer has been widely accepted across the world to decrease the risk and incidence of multifetal pregnancy, without any significant reduction in the cumulative pregnancy rate.[27] With the improvement of the field of embryology, the percentage of blastocyst culture and blastocyst transfer has increased. Blastocyst transfer is associated with increased implantation rate and pregnancy rate when compared to cleavage stage embryo transfer.[28,29] Therefore, single blastocyst transfer can be advocated in women with chronic hypertension.

Therefore, in patients with chronic hypertension, mild ovarian stimulation (appropriate), use of letrozole along with gonadotropin, fresh embryo transfer (in case of poor responders or patients with a low risk of OHSS), natural cycle/stimulated cycle FET, and single embryo transfer may be advocated to prevent worsening of the hypertension and to prevent morbidity. However, good quality studies dealing with patients who have chronic hypertension are needed to derive robust conclusion.

■ OBSTETRIC CONCERNS IN HYPERTENSIVE DISORDERS

Chronic hypertension is a risk factor for preeclampsia. IVF is also a risk factor for eclampsia. Therefore, women with chronic hypertension undergoing IVF treatment are at a higher risk of developing eclampsia/preeclampsia.

Once the pregnancy is achieved, special precautions have to be taken to prevent preeclampsia. Use of low-dose aspirin has been recommended by World Health Organization (WHO), American College of Obstetricians and Gynecologists (ACOG), and Royal College of Obstetricians and Gynaecologists (RCOG). WHO along with ACOG recommends the initiation of low-dose aspirin (at a dose of 75 mg or above) to prevent eclampsia.[30]

BOX 3: Investigations for baseline evaluation of chronic hypertension before pregnancy.

- Serum aspartate aminotransferase and alanine aminotransferase
- Serum creatinine
- Serum electrolytes (specifically potassium)
- Blood urea nitrogen
- Complete blood count
- Spot urine protein/creatinine ratio or 24-hour urine for total protein and creatinine (to calculate creatinine clearance) as appropriate
- Electrocardiogram or echocardiogram as appropriate

Low-dose aspirin should be started from 12 weeks and preferably not later than 16 weeks of gestation.

In patients who have chronic hypertension, preeclampsia has an earlier onset and usually tends to be more severe. Moreover, the prognosis for the woman and fetus is worse than preeclampsia alone. Therefore, stringent monitoring of the patient's clinical aspect is required. More frequent prenatal visits (every 2-4 weeks if blood pressure is well controlled and weekly if blood pressure is not well controlled) are recommended compared with healthy women. Such visits are designed to evaluate women for complications of chronic hypertension in pregnancy by following blood pressures, urine protein, fundal height, and maternal symptoms.

Box 3 demonstrates the tests that are recommended by All India Congress of Obstetrics & Gynaecology (AICOG) for baseline evaluation of a pregnant woman having chronic hypertension.

Antepartum fetal surveillance is quite essential to reduce perinatal morbidity and mortality in pregnant women who have chronic hypertension. Since chronic hypertension is a risk factor of developing preeclampsia, pregnant hypertensive women who conceive through ART should be categorically screened for preeclampsia. A new algorithm combining maternal uterine artery resistance measured by Doppler ultrasound, mean arterial blood pressure, and circulating placental growth factor (PlGF) levels has been proposed. This test has been reported to be superior in predicting preterm preeclampsia when compared to clinical risk factors alone.[31] It has been demonstrated that this has a detection rate of 82% of the cases, which is double of that achieved by applying clinical factors using National Institute for Health and Care Excellence (NICE) guidelines.[32]

Since patients with chronic hypertension have increased risks of fetal growth restriction, third-trimester ultrasound assessment of fetal growth and subsequent evaluation are required as appropriate. Fetal growth restriction surveillance should be done at 2-4 weeks' interval starting from the third trimester and depending on blood pressure, complications, medications, and findings in prior scans. No single protocol is demonstrated

Flowchart 1: Severe preeclampsia management algorithm.

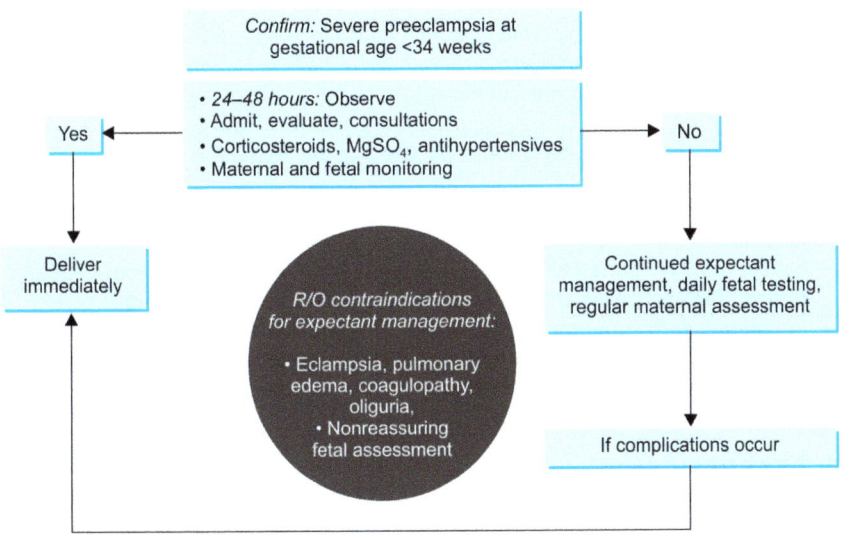

to be superior in utility than others; testing often includes daily fetal kick counts, fetal heart rate testing (i.e., nonstress testing), and ultrasound evaluation of amniotic fluid volume or fetal tone and movements (part of biophysical profile). Women with severe preeclampsia should deliver by 34 weeks **(Flowchart 1)**. In women with superimposed preeclampsia without severe features and with stable maternal and fetal conditions, expectant management until 37 0/7 weeks of gestation with close maternal and fetal surveillance is suggested. In women with chronic hypertension, who require no medications, delivery can be recommended between 38 and 39 weeks of gestation.

Postnatal follow-up should be done daily for the first 2 days after delivery and at least once between the third day and fifth day after birth. Antihypertensive may be changed if clinically indicated. Two weeks after delivery, the patient must review with the cardiologist for clinical assessment and antihypertensive optimization.

■ CONCLUSION

Women with chronic hypertension needs proper preconception care to optimize their health before IVF. Single blastocyst transfer can minimize the risk of multiple pregnancy and thereby the risk of preeclampsia. Low dose aspirin should be used as prophylaxis for high-risk cases. During pregnancy, maternal and fetal parameters should be carefully monitored. In case of superimposed preeclampsia, timing of delivery should be optimized.

KEY LEARNING POINTS

- Proper preconception counseling should be done; medication should be altered and blood pressure optimized.
- IVF should be tailored to prevent increase in serum estradiol and to reduce the risk of OHSS.
- Single blastocyst transfer should be tried to decrease the risk of multifetal pregnancy.
- If the patient is undergoing FET, natural cycle or stimulated cycle FET must be targeted.
- Patient must be started with low-dose aspirin and low-molecular-weight heparin during the luteal phase or latest when the pregnancy test comes positive.
- In patients with superimposed preeclampsia, without severe features and with stable maternal and fetal conditions, expectant management until 37 0/7 weeks of gestation with close maternal and fetal surveillance is suggested.

■ REFERENCES

1. Bramham K, Parnell B, Nelson-Piercy C, Seed PT, Poston L, Chappell LC. Chronic hypertension and pregnancy outcomes: systematic review and meta-analysis. BMJ. 2014;348:g2301.
2. Dayan N, Lanes A, Walker MC, Spitzer KA, Laskin CA. Effect of chronic hypertension on assisted pregnancy outcomes: a population-based study in Ontario, Canada. Fertil Steril. 2016;105(4):1003-9.
3. Banerjee K. IVF in medically complicated patient—a review. AOGD Bull. 2019;19(3):37.
4. Guo D, Li S, Behr B, Eisenberg ML. Hypertension and male fertility. World J Mens Health. 2017;35(2):59-64.
5. American College of Obstetricians and Gynecologists. ACOG Practice Bulletin No. 125: chronic hypertension in pregnancy. Obstet Gynecol. 2012;119(2 Pt 1):396-407.
6. Carson MP, Chen KK. Hypertension in a woman planning pregnancy. CMAJ. 2014;186(2):129-30.
7. Zhou A, Xiong C, Hu R, Zhang Y, Bassig BA, Triche E, et al. Pre-pregnancy BMI, gestational weight gain, and the risk of hypertensive disorders of pregnancy: a cohort study in Wuhan, China. PLoS One. 2015;10(8):e0136291.
8. Hall JE, do Carmo JM, da Silva AA, Wang Z, Hall ME. Obesity-induced hypertension: interaction of neurohumoral and renal mechanisms. Circ Res. 2015;116(6):991-1006.
9. Graudal NA, Hubeck-Graudal T, Jurgens G. Effects of low sodium diet versus high sodium diet on blood pressure, renin, aldosterone, catecholamines, cholesterol, and triglyceride. Cochrane Database Syst Rev. 2020;12(12):CD004022.
10. Tang N, Ma J, Tao R, Chen Z, Yang Y, He Q, et al. The effects of the interaction between BMI and dyslipidemia on hypertension in adults. Sci Rep. 2022;12(1):1-7.
11. Benoff S, Cooper GW, Hurley I, Mandel FS, Rosenfeld DL, Scholl GM, et al. The effect of calcium ion channel blockers on sperm fertilization potential. Fertil Steril. 1994;62(3):606-17.
12. Sunkara SK, Rittenberg V, Raine-Fenning N, Bhattacharya S, Zamora J, Coomarasamy A. Association between the number of eggs and live birth

in IVF treatment: an analysis of 400 135 treatment cycles. Human Reprod. 2011;26(7):1768-74.
13. Dobrosavljevic A, Rakic S. Risk of gestational hypertension in pregnancies complicated with ovarian hyperstimulation syndrome. J Pak Med Assoc. 2020;70(11):1897-1900.
14. Agbabiaka AA, D'Angelo A. The use of frozen embryo transfer and the development of pregnancy-induced hypertension: a literature review. EMJ Reprod Health. 2021;7(1):44-53.
15. Gu F, Wu Y, Tan M, Hu R, Chen Y, Li X, et al. Programmed frozen embryo transfer cycle increased risk of hypertensive disorders of pregnancy: a multicenter cohort study in ovulatory women. Am J Obstet Gynecol MFM. 2023;5(1):100752.
16. Shi Y, Sun Y, Hao C, Zhang H, Wei D, Zhang Y, et al. Transfer of fresh versus frozen embryos in ovulatory women. N Engl J Med. 2018;378(2):126-36.
17. Liu C, Li Y, Jiang H, Liu Y, Song X. The clinical outcomes of fresh versus frozen embryos transfer in women ≥40 years with poor ovarian response. Obstet Gynecol Sci. 2021;64(3):284-92.
18. Oktay K, Hourvitz A, Sahin G, Oktem O, Safro B, Cil A, et al. Letrozole reduces estrogen and gonadotropin exposure in women with breast cancer undergoing ovarian stimulation before chemotherapy. J Clin Endocrinol Metab. 2006;91(10):3885-90.
19. Haas J, Bassil R, Meriano J, Samara N, Barzilay E, Gonen N, et al. Does daily co-administration of letrozole and gonadotropins during ovarian stimulation improve IVF outcome? Reprod Biol Endocrinol. 2017;15:70.
20. Bülow NS, Skouby SO, Warzecha AK, Udengaard H, Andersen CY, Holt MD, et al. Impact of letrozole co-treatment during ovarian stimulation with gonadotrophins for IVF: a multicentre, randomized, double-blinded placebo-controlled trial. Hum Reprod. 2022;37(2):309-21.
21. Bortoletto P, Prabhu M, Baker VL. Association between programmed frozen embryo transfer and hypertensive disorders of pregnancy. Fertil Steril. 2022;118(5):839-48.
22. Singh B, Reschke L, Segars J, Baker VL. Frozen-thawed embryo transfer: the potential importance of the corpus luteum in preventing obstetrical complications. Fertil Steril. 2020;113(2):252-7.
23. Saito K, Kuwahara A, Ishikawa T, Morisaki N, Miyado M, Miyado K, et al. Endometrial preparation methods for frozen-thawed embryo transfer are associated with altered risks of hypertensive disorders of pregnancy, placenta accreta, and gestational diabetes mellitus. Human Reprod. 2019;34(8):1567-75.
24. Ernstad EG, Wennerholm UB, Khatibi A, Petzold M, Bergh C. Neonatal and maternal outcome after frozen embryo transfer: increased risks in programmed cycles. Am J Obstet Gynecol. 2019;221(2):126.e1.
25. Zong L, Liu P, Zhou L, Wei D, Ding L, Qin Y. Increased risk of maternal and neonatal complications in hormone replacement therapy cycles in frozen embryo transfer. Reprod Biol Endocrinol. 2020;18(1):36.
26. Krotz S, Fajardo J, Ghandi S, Patel A, Keith LG. Hypertensive disease in twin pregnancies: a review. Twin Res Hum Genet. 2002;5(1):8-14.
27. Kamath MS, Mascarenhas M, Kirubakaran R, Bhattacharya S. Number of embryos for transfer following in vitro fertilisation or intra-cytoplasmic sperm injection. Cochrane Database Syst Rev. 2020;8(8):CD003416.

28. Glujovsky D, Retamar AM, Sedo CR, Ciapponi A, Cornelisse S, Blake D. Cleavage-stage versus blastocyst-stage embryo transfer in assisted reproductive technology. Cochrane Database Syst Rev. 2022;5(5):CD002118.
29. Practice Committee of the American Society for Reproductive Medicine, Practice Committee of the Society for Assisted Reproductive Technology. Blastocyst culture and transfer in clinically assisted reproduction: a committee opinion. Fertil Steril. 2018;110(7):1246-52.
30. American College of Obstetricians and Gynecologists. ACOG committee opinion no. 743: low-dose aspirin use during pregnancy. Obstet Gynecol. 2018;132(1):e44-52.
31. MacDonald TM, Walker SP, Hannan NJ, Tong S, Kaitu'u-Lino TJ. Clinical tools and biomarkers to predict preeclampsia. EBioMedicine. 2022;75:103780.
32. Tan MY, Wright D, Syngelaki A, Akolekar R, Cicero S, Janga D, et al. Comparison of diagnostic accuracy of early screening for pre-eclampsia by NICE guidelines and a method combining maternal factors and biomarkers: results of SPREE. Ultrasound Obstet Gynecol. 2018;51(6):743-50.

17

Fertility and Assisted Reproductive Technology in Diabetes Mellitus

Sweta Gupta, Puja Kumari, Preyander Singh Thakur

■ INTRODUCTION

The global diabetes prevalence in 2019 is estimated to be 9.3% (463 million people), rising to 10.2% (578 million) by 2030 and 10.9% (700 million) by 2045. The prevalence is higher in urban (10.8%) than rural (7.2%) areas and in high-income (10.4%) than low-income countries (4.0%).[1]

With advancement of childbearing age and exponential increase in prevalence of diabetes, now more and more number of women desiring fertility are presenting with either frank diabetes or prediabetes, complicating the fertility options further. Well-balanced diet and regular physical activity help to maintain normal body weight and prevent the onset of type 2 diabetes mellitus (T2DM). Diabetes can be controlled, and regular screening and its treatment can avoid complications and consequences. This chapter shall focus on special needs of these women in reproductive age group.

■ DIABETES AND ITS EFFECT ON FERTILITY

Reproductive health problems in women with diabetes range from delayed puberty, delayed menarche, menstrual cycle irregularities, subfertility, adverse pregnancy and neonatal outcome, and early menopause.[2]

Poorly controlled type 1 diabetes mellitus (T1DM) women frequently have hypothalamic amenorrhea and subfertility, otherwise fertility is usually normal in women with T1DM.[3] Similarly, age of menopause is also normal in most of the women with T1DM; however, in rare instances, autoimmune premature ovarian insufficiency can coexist with diabetes **(Box 1)**.

There is a "U-shaped" relationship among menarche, menopause, and T2DM, with both early and late menarche/menopause being risk factors for

BOX 1: Infertility risk factors related to diabetes mellitus in women.

- Menstrual abnormalities
- Shortening of reproductive period (late menarche and premature menopause)
- Poor glycemic control and presence of diabetes complications
- Hyperandrogenism and polycystic ovary syndrome
- Autoimmunity (Hashimoto's thyroiditis)
- Sexual dysfunction

BOX 2: Infertility risk factors related to diabetes mellitus in men.

- Reduced sperm count and motility
- Impairment of spermatogenesis
- *Male subfertility:* Altered steroidogenesis
- Epigenetic dysregulation in spermatogenesis
- Impairment in sperm DNA integrity
- Erectile dysfunction
- Decreased testosterone concentration (hypogonadism)

(DNA: deoxyribonucleic acid)

T2DM, according to the literature on the subject of T2DM and the female reproductive lifespan, menstrual cycle disorders, fertility problems, and gestational health in women with T2DM.[4]

Similarly, in men, both T1DM and T2DM can lead to subfertility **(Box 2)**.[5]

■ PRECONCEPTION COUNSELING AND WORK-UP

Optimizing Glycemic Control

Reproductive age women with diabetes should be informed and counseled about the importance of achieving of euglycemia prior to conception and throughout pregnancy. In order to lower the risk of congenital abnormalities, preeclampsia, macrosomia, and other fetal and maternal issues, preconception counseling should emphasize the significance of maintaining glucose levels near to normal, with the optimal glycated hemoglobin (HbA1c) being 6.5% (48 mmol/mol) **(Box 3)**.[6]

There is an increased risk of diabetic embryopathy, especially neural tube defects, congenital heart disease, renal anomalies, and caudal dysgenesis, which are directly proportional to elevations in HbA1c during the first 10 weeks of pregnancy. The absolute risk of congenital anomaly in a newborn is approximately 3% (similar to general population) when preconception HbA1c is <6.7% to as high as 10% with HbA1c of >11.3%.[7]

Therefore, where possible, preconception care for pregnant women with preexisting diabetes should begin in a multidisciplinary clinic comprising an endocrinologist, maternal–fetal medicine specialist, registered dietitian nutritionist, and diabetes educator.[6]

The risk of developing and/or progressing diabetic retinopathy as well as diabetic nephropathy should be discussed with women who have preexisting T1DM or T2DM and are contemplating on becoming pregnant or who have already been pregnant. Therefore, eye examinations should occur ideally before pregnancy or in the first trimester, and then patients should be monitored every trimester and for 1 year postpartum as indicated by the degree of retinopathy and as recommended by the eye care provider.[6]

BOX 3: Fetal, neonatal, and maternal complications associated with diabetes in pregnancy.

Fetal
- Miscarriage
- Intrauterine death/stillbirth/preterm labor
- Congenital anomalies [vertebral defects, anal atresia, cardiac defects, tracheoesophageal fistula, renal and limb abnormalities (VACTERL)]
- Macrosomia
- Shoulder dystocia/brachial plexus injury

Newborn
- Hypoglycemia
- Hypomagnesemia, hypocalcemia, hyperbilirubinemia
- Polycythemia
- Respiratory distress syndrome
- Transient hypertrophic cardiomyopathy
- Birth asphyxia

Maternal
- Increased chances of cesarean section
- Preeclampsia/eclampsia
- Increased risk of postpartum hemorrhage (both traumatic and atonic)
- Increased risk of purpureal/wound sepsis

BOX 4: Drugs to be withheld before or immediately after conception.

- All oral antidiabetic drugs except for metformin and glyburide in exceptional cases
- All injectable antidiabetic drugs except for insulin
- ACE inhibitors
- Statins
- Beta-blockers

(ACE: angiotensin-converting enzyme)

Similarly, urine protein excretion as well as serum creatinine measurement should be conducted before conception and at least once in each trimester.

For women with T2DM on oral or noninsulin injectable agents, consider change to insulin prior to pregnancy, even in women with good glycemic control. Patients should be counseled regarding the possible need of insulin changes and withholding teratogenic drugs such as statins and angiotensin-converting enzyme (ACE) inhibitors during pregnancy **(Box 4)**. The patient should be ideally switched over to a basal–bolus insulin regimen, i.e., three times premeal boluses of short-acting insulin and once- or twice-daily basal long-acting insulin.

Screening for sexually transmitted diseases and thyroid diseases, recommended vaccinations, and routine genetic screening should be done as standard protocol.

Prior to conception, it is advised to take prenatal vitamins that contain at least 400 mg of folic acid and 150 g of potassium iodide.[8]

In order to lower the incidence of preeclampsia, aspirin (81–150 mg) should be used by all diabetic pregnant women by 16 weeks of gestation (if there are no contraindications).[9]

Glycemic Targets

The American Diabetes Association (ADA) and the American Association of Clinical Endocrinologists (AACE) recommend the following targets for women with T1DM or T2DM, similar to the targets recommended by the American College of Obstetricians and Gynecologists (ACOG) [which are the same as for gestational diabetes mellitus (GDM), outlined below]:[10]

- Fasting blood glucose 5.3 mmol/L or below, and either
- Blood sugar <140 mg/dL (7.8 mmol/L) 1 hour after eating or
- 2-hour postprandial glucose level of <120 mg/dL (6.7 mmol/L).

Diet and Exercise

The best dietary strategy for glycemic management, especially in instances of T1DM, involves careful carbohydrate counting. If at all possible, the team should include a qualified dietician or certified diabetes educator. Particularly in women who are on several daily insulin injections, meals should be separated into a three-meal and three-snacks pattern (breakfast, lunch, supper, midmorning snack, evening snack, and late-night snack).

Dietary recommendations include 40–50% complex, high-fiber carbs, 15–30% protein, and 20–35% unsaturated fats.

Trans fats should be avoided, and saturated fats should not exceed 10%.

Typical carbohydrate breakdown:
- *Breakfast:* 30–45 g, lunch and dinner: 45–60 g, snacks: 15 g snacks every 2–3 hours
- *Exercise:* At least 30 minutes of light aerobic exercise on at least 5 days per week.

Optimal weight: Body mass index (BMI) >20 to <25 kg/m^2 is recommended. Patients should be counseled to avoid use of nicotine products, alcohol, and recreational drugs, including marijuana.

Endocrinologist Review

A review by an endocrinologist is required for complete assessment to have optimal diabetic control with minimum complications.

SPECIAL CARE TO BE TAKEN DURING FERTILITY TREATMENT AND IN VITRO FERTILIZATION

Ovarian hyperstimulation syndrome can occur in patients who receive gonadotropins for ovarian stimulation during in vitro fertilization (IVF) cycles. T2DM and the morphology of polycystic ovary syndrome (PCOS) are significant risk factors that increase the incidence of ovarian hyperstimulation. PCOS is more frequently observed in people with diabetes or prediabetes. Patients with T2DM frequently experience hyperinsulinemia brought on by insulin resistance. The risk of ovarian hyperstimulation during IVF is increased overall as a result of this hyperinsulinemia, which in turn causes hyperestrogenemia.

Metformin has a positive effect on the prevention of such issues among diabetic females pursuing IVF pregnancy as demonstrated in multiple research. Estradiol concentrations are decreased as a result of metformin-induced reductions in androgen and insulin levels. Furthermore, evidence points to metformin's distinct influence on human ovarian steroidogenesis.

Moreover, metformin has also been shown to directly suppress the activity of aromatase enzyme.[11-15]

Precautions during Oocyte Pickup

The diabetic patient should be handled as the first patient in the morning as a precaution during oocyte pickup (OPU). No oral or noninsulin injectable antidiabetic medications should be given on the day of surgery, according to the consensus statement on blood glucose management from the Society for Ambulatory Anesthesia (SAMBA). These medications should not be stopped the day before surgery, though. SAMBA advises delaying the introduction of postsurgical oral and noninsulin injectable treatment regimens until after returning to a regular diet. On the morning of surgery, short-acting or rapid-acting insulin should not be administered, according to all professional organizations. The anesthesia provider should recommend a short-acting or rapid-acting insulin dose in the event of awakening hyperglycemia. Taking long-acting insulin, which is typically dosed at bedtime, should be 75-100% of the usual dose. SAMBA generally recommends that a blood glucose level of <180 mg/dL (10.0 mmol/L) is optimal for the ambulatory office setting because postoperative hypoglycemia and hyperglycemia are associated with poor patient outcomes. Blood glucose levels must be monitored after surgery and anesthesia.[16]

Assisted Reproductive Technology Outcome in Diabetes

Assisted reproductive technology (ART) outcomes are also poorer in women with T2DM compared to either healthy subjects or those having T1DM.

A large cohort study aimed to examine the chance of biochemical pregnancy, clinical pregnancy, and live birth after ART treatment in women with T1DM and T2DM, comprising 594 women with either T1DM or T2DM, found that relative to women without diabetes, chances of live birth per embryo transfer were reduced by 50% in women with T2DM and were almost similar in women with T1DM.[17]

Assisted Reproductive Technology and Risk of Gestational Diabetes Mellitus

A recently published meta-analysis has shown that women who gave birth through ART have a 53% increased risk of gestational diabetes compared to women who conceived naturally.[18]

WHAT PRECAUTIONS SHOULD BE TAKEN DURING PREGNANCY AND IN NEONATES?

Glycemic targets should be optimal before planning pregnancy. Multidisciplinary input of endocrinologist, fertility specialist, dietician, counselor, and obstetrician should be taken in **(Box 5)**. Neonates born to diabetic mothers should be observed closely for complications mentioned in **Box 3**.

Aspirin should be started by 12–16 weeks to reduce the risk of preeclampsia.

Type 1 Diabetes Mellitus and Hypothyroidism

Patients with T1DM frequently have thyroid issues that also must be controlled. Up to 30–40% of young women with T1DM have thyroid disease too, and women with T1DM have a 5–10% risk of developing autoimmune thyroid disease first diagnosed in pregnancy (most commonly Hashimoto's thyroiditis).[19]

As the fetus is completely dependent on maternal thyroid hormone in the first trimester, thyroid stimulating hormone (TSH) should be checked prior to pregnancy and at least once during each trimester.[20,21]

Patients having T2DM should also be routinely screened for thyroid disorders during pregnancy as there is an increased incidence of thyroid disorders in patients with T2DM also.[22]

BOX 5: Precautions to be taken during pregnancy in diabetes.

- Frequent self-monitoring of blood glucose and to adhere to glycemic targets
- Swift titration of insulin dosage whenever indicated
- To follow medical nutrition therapy
- Adhere to predefined exercise program
- Regular obstetric checkups, including USG scans

(USG: ultrasonography)

Type 2 Diabetes Mellitus and Cardiovascular Comorbidity

Women with T2DM are commonly associated with dyslipidemia and hypertension. Chronic hypertension occurs in 13-19% of women with T2DM, and many of these will be prescribed an ACE inhibitor or angiotensin receptor blocker (ARB).[23] The benefits and hazards of quitting these medications before becoming pregnant must be discussed in detail depending on the indication for usage, but they should be stopped immediately after a missed period. The data on teratogenicity of statins for the treatment of hypercholesterolemia is also conflicting and is based on animal, not human, studies.[24] Pravastatin has shown favorable effects on vascular endothelial growth factor in animal studies.[25,26] However, at this time, the current guidelines recommend that statins be stopped prior to pregnancy.

Effects of Pregnancy on Diabetes

Early pregnancy is a time of enhanced insulin sensitivity and lower glucose levels. Many women with T1DM will have lower insulin requirements and hence may have an increased risk for hypoglycemia.[27] The situation rapidly reverses by approximately 16 weeks as insulin resistance subsequently increases to its highest level in the third trimester.

Insulin Use

The ADA and ACOG recommend insulin as the first-line agent for the treatment of diabetes in pregnancy, including preexisting diabetes and GDM. Insulin therapy must be individualized for women with preexisting diabetes in pregnancy.

Insulin is the preferred agent for the management of both T1DM and T2DM in pregnancy.
- Either multiple daily injections or insulin pump technology can be used in pregnancy complicated by T1DM.
- The physiology of pregnancy necessitates frequent titration of insulin to match changing requirements and underscores the importance of daily and frequent self-monitoring of blood glucose. Due to the complexity of insulin management in pregnancy, referral to a specialized center offering team-based care (with team members including maternal-fetal medicine specialist, endocrinologist, or other providers experienced in managing pregnancy in women with preexisting diabetes, dietitian, nurse, and social worker, as needed) is recommended.

In patients, if corticosteroids are administered to accelerate lung maturation in the setting of an obstetric complication, an increased insulin requirement during the next 5 days should be anticipated, and the patient's glucose levels should be closely monitored.[10]

Metformin Use During Pregnancy

The use of metformin has been found to be safe in pregnancy in a large trial (MiG trial) where it was compared with insulin.[28] However, its subsequent follow-up study, i.e., MiG-TOFU, has shown some concerns with higher BMI being reported in children born to mothers who were on metformin during their gestation.[29] However, this follow-up study should be taken with a pinch of salt as most of the subjects were lost to follow-up leading to underpowering of the study. Another study which is currently undergoing, the Metformin in Women with Type 2 Diabetes in Pregnancy Trial (MiTy), shall help in clearing the picture further. Till then, metformin can be used cautiously, especially in second and third trimesters, wherever indicated, especially in resource-poor countries such as India where stringent follow-up may be difficult.[30]

Management of Hypoglycemia

Any blood glucose level <70 mg/dL during pregnancy should be classified as hypoglycemia. When signs of hypoglycemia such as tremors, palpitations, hunger, or excessive perspiration arise, blood sugar levels should be examined very away. A condition known as the Somogyi phenomenon occurs when nocturnal hypoglycemia (low blood sugar between 2 and 3 AM) is occasionally missed, and greater values of fasting blood sugar are measured the next morning as a result of the release of counterregulatory hormones. To combat this occurrence, the dose of basal insulin should be decreased rather than increased, and a sufficient bedtime snack should be provided.

Glucose Monitoring Timing and Frequency

Tight glycemic control should be achieved by frequent self-monitoring of glucose by pregnant diabetic women. As fetal macrosomia (overgrowth) is related to increased fasting and postprandial glucose levels, pregnant women with diabetes need to monitor their pre- and postmeal and fasting glucose levels regularly.[31] Patients should be followed and assessed every 1-2 weeks during the first two trimesters and every week after 24-28 weeks.

Continuous Glucose Monitoring

Continuous glucose monitoring (CGM) can be used as an adjunctive therapy with self-monitored blood glucose (SMBG) values in patients with frequent or severe hypoglycemia during pregnancy.

It may be used in conjunction with an insulin pump or with metered dose inhaler (MDI) therapy to help achieve glycemic control. The continuous glucose monitoring in pregnant women with type 1 diabetes (CONCEPTT) trial was a large multicenter trial that examined CGM use in women and found a statistically significantly lower incidence of large for gestational age

(LGA) infants, less neonatal intensive care unit stays for >24 hours, and less neonatal hypoglycemia.[32] Various CGM devices available in the market are currently expensive and hence cannot be prescribed to every patient.

■ CONCLUSION

Diabetes effects both reproductive men and women. It is important to have proper assessment at the time of preconception period. Individualized multidisciplinary approach for both diabetes and fertility wellbeing are required for best outcome in relation to fertility, pregnancy, and neonatal period.

KEY LEARNING POINTS

Key points for care during fertility treatment in a diabetic patient:
- Success rates of treatment are similar to those obtained in women who do not have diabetes if all necessary care is taken. The type of fertility treatment will depend on age, duration of infertility, cause of infertility, and basic investigations such as semen analysis, anti-Müllerian hormone (AMH), and tubal patency.
- Organogenesis takes place following transfer and during the first few weeks of pregnancy. Following transfer and throughout the first few weeks of pregnancy, organogenesis occurs. Diabetes metabolic regulation is essential during that time to lower the risk of congenital malformations and miscarriage.
- HBA1c levels should be as close to normal (<6.5) as possible before planning pregnancy.
- Lifestyle modification is an important part of the management of GDM and may suffice for the treatment of many women. To achieve glycemic targets, insulin can be added if required.
- Insulin is the medication of choice for treatment of hyperglycemia in GDM for those who are unable to achieve the euglycemic level by medical nutrition therapy. Metformin and glyburide should be used judiciously in selected patients only with caution.

■ REFERENCES

1. Saeedi P, Petersohn I, Salpea P, Malanda B, Karuranga S, Unwin N, et al. Global and regional diabetes prevalence estimates for 2019 and projections for 2030 and 2045: results from the International Diabetes Federation Diabetes Atlas, 9th edition. Diabetes Res Clin Pract. 2019;157:107843.
2. Thong EP, Codner E, Laven JSE, Teede H. Diabetes: a metabolic and reproductive disorder in women. Lancet Diabetes Endocrinol. 2020;8(2):134-49.
3. Holt RIG, Cockram C, Flyvbjerg A, Goldstein BJ. Textbook of Diabetes, 5th edition. New Jersey: Wiley-Blackwell; 2017.
4. Crețu D, Cernea S, Onea CR, Pop RM. Reproductive health in women with type 2 diabetes mellitus. Hormones (Athens). 2020;19(3):291-300.
5. Ding GL, Liu Y, Liu ME, Pan JX, Guo MX, Sheng JZ, et al. The effects of diabetes on male fertility and epigenetic regulation during spermatogenesis. Asian J Androl. 2015;17(6):948-53.

6. American Diabetes Association. Standards of Care in Diabetes—2023 abridged for primary care providers. Clin Diabetes. 2023;41(1):4-31.
7. Guerin A, Nisenbaum R, Ray JG. Use of maternal GHb concentration to estimate the risk of congenital anomalies in the offspring of women with prepregnancy diabetes. Diabetes Care. 2007;30(7):120-5.
8. Alexander EK, Pearce EN, Brent GA, Brown RS, Chen H, Dosiou C, et al. 2017 guidelines of the American Thyroid Association for the diagnosis and management of thyroid disease during pregnancy and the post-partum. Thyroid. 2017;27:315-89.
9. Henderson JT, Whitlock EP, O'Conner E, Senger CA, Thompson JH, Rowland MG. Low-dose aspirin for the prevention of morbidity and mortality from preeclampsia: a systematic evidence review for the U.S. Preventive Services Task Force, 2014. Ann Intern Med. 2014;160(10):695-703.
10. American College of Obstetricians and Gynecologists' Committee on Practice Bulletins: Obstetrics. ACOG Practice Bulletin No. 201: Pregestational Diabetes Mellitus. Obstet Gynecol. 2018;132(6):e228-48.
11. Tang T, Glanville J, Orsi N, Barth JH, Balen AH. The use of metformin for women with PCOS undergoing IVF treatment. Hum Reprod. 2006;21(6):1416-25.
12. Haas DA, Carr BR, Attia GR. Effects of metformin on body mass index, menstrual cyclicity, and ovulation induction in women with polycystic ovary syndrome. Fertil Steril. 2003;79(3):469-81.
13. Harborne L, Fleming R, Lyall H, Norman J, Sattar N. Descriptive review of the evidence for the use of metformin in polycystic ovary syndrome. Lancet. 2003;361(9372):1894-901.
14. Kjøtrød SB, von Düring V, Carlsen SM. Metformin treatment before IVF/ICSI in women with polycystic ovary syndrome; a prospective, randomized, double blind study. Hum Reprod. 2004;19(6):1315-22.
15. Mansfield R, Galea R, Brincat M, Hole D, Mason H. Metformin has direct effects on human ovarian steroidogenesis. Fertil Steril. 2003;79(4):956-62.
16. Cornelius BW. Patients with type 2 diabetes: anesthetic management in the ambulatory setting: part 2: pharmacology and guidelines for perioperative management. Anesth Prog. 2017;64(1):39-44.
17. Larsen MD, Jensen DM, Fedder J, Jølving LR, Nørgård BM. Live-born children after assisted reproduction in women with type 1 diabetes and type 2 diabetes: a nationwide cohort study. Diabetologia. 2020;63(9):1736-44.
18. Anagnostis P, et al. Abstract 921. Presented at European Association for the Study of Diabetes Annual Meeting, September 16-20, 2019, Barcelona, Spain.
19. Umpierrez GE, Latif KA, Murphy MB, Lambeth HC, Stentz F, Bush A, et al. Thyroid dysfunction in patients with type 1 diabetes: a longitudinal study. Diabetes Care. 2003;26(4):1181-5.
20. Stagnaro-Green A, Abalovich M, Alexander E, Azizi F, Mestman J, Negro R, et al. Guidelines of the American Thyroid Association for the diagnosis and management of thyroid disease during pregnancy and postpartum. Thyroid. 2011;21(10):1081-125.
21. Gonzalez-Gonzalez NL, Ramirez O, Mozas J, Melchor J, Armas H, Garcia-Hernandez JA, et al. Factors influencing pregnancy outcome in women with type 2 versus type 1 diabetes mellitus. Acta Obstet Gynecol Scand. 2008;87(1):43-9.

22. Kalra S, Aggarwal S, Khandelwal D. Thyroid dysfunction and type 2 diabetes mellitus: screening strategies and implications for management. Diabetes Ther. 2019;10(6):2035-44.
23. Kazmin A, Garcia-Bournissen F, Koren G. Risks of statin use during pregnancy: a systematic review. J Obstet Gynaecol Can. 2007;29(11):906-8.
24. Cudmore M, Ahmad S, Al-Ani B, Fujisawa T, Coxall H, Chudasama K, et al. Negative regulation of soluble Flt-1 and soluble endoglin release by heme oxygenase-1. Circulation. 2007;115(13):1789-97.
25. Costantine MM, Cleary K. Pravastatin for the prevention of preeclampsia in high-risk pregnant women. Obstet Gynecol. 2013;121:349-53.
26. Costantine MM, Tamayo E, Lu F, Bytautiene E, Longo M, Hankins GDV, et al. Using pravastatin to improve the vascular reactivity in a mouse model of soluble fms-like tyrosine kinase-1-induced preeclampsia. Obstet Gynecol. 2010;116(1):114-20.
27. Garcia-Patterson A, Gich I, Amini SB, Catalano PM, de Leiva A, Corcoy R. Insulin requirements throughout pregnancy in women with type 1 diabetes mellitus: three changes of direction. Diabetologia. 2010;53:44651.
28. Rowan JA, Hague WM, Gao W, Battin MR, Moore MP, MiG Trial Investigators. Metformin versus insulin for the treatment of gestational diabetes. N Engl J Med. 2008;358(19):2003-15.
29. Rowan JA, Rush EC, Plank LD, Lu J, Obolonkin V, Coat S, et al. Metformin in gestational diabetes: the offspring follow-up (MiG TOFU): body composition and metabolic outcomes at 7-9 years of age. BMJ Open Diabetes Res Care. 2018;6(1):e000456.
30. Feig DS, Murphy K, Asztalos E, Tomlinson G, Sanchez J, Zinman B, et al. Metformin in women with type 2 diabetes in pregnancy (MiTy): a multi-center randomized controlled trial. BMC Pregnancy Childbirth. 2016;16(1):173.
31. de Veciana M, Major CA, Morgan MA, Asrat T, Toohey JS, Lien JM, et al. Postprandial versus preprandial blood glucose monitoring in women with gestational diabetes mellitus requiring insulin therapy. N Engl J Med. 1995;333(19):1237-41.
32. Feig DS, Donovan LE, Corcoy R, Murphy KE, Amiel SA, Hunt KF, et al. Continuous glucose monitoring in pregnant women with type 1 diabetes (CONCEPTT): a multicentre international randomised controlled trial. Lancet. 2017;390: 2347-59.

Index

Page numbers followed by *b* refer to box, *f* refer to figure, *fc* refer to flowchart, and *t* refer to table.

A

Abortion, spontaneous 93
Abruption 125
Acetylsalicylic acid 103
Adriamycin 74
Alanine aminotransferase 136
Aldosterone receptor blockers 3
Alkaline phosphatase 136
Alpha-fetoprotein 136
Amenorrhea 93
　chemotherapy-related 34
　treatment-induced 33
Anal atresia 159
Anemia 15, 89
　autoimmune hemolytic 95
Angiotensin-converting enzyme 159
　inhibitors 148, 159
Angiotensin-receptor blockers 148, 163
Antepartum fetal surveillance 152
Anticoagulant 99
　therapy 100
Antihypertensives 3, 148*b*
Anti-Müllerian hormone 21, 33, 47, 85, 109, 118
Antiphospholipid syndrome 102, 103
Antithrombin deficiency, hereditary 103
Apixaban 100
Artificial ovary 65
Aspartate aminotransferase 136
Assisted reproductive technology 2, 10, 13, 32, 36, 46, 54, 57, 61, 65, 77, 82, 92, 95, 99, 107, 108*f*, 110, 115, 131, 146, 149, 157, 161, 162
　complications of 124
Atenolol 148
Autoimmune disease 92, 95
Autoimmune disorders 92
Autoimmunity 92, 157
Autonomic dysfunction 74
Autotransplantation 64
Azathioprine 12
Azoospermia
　nonobstructive 77
　obstructive 77

B

Bariatric surgery 83, 85, 86, 89
　effect of 85*t*
Beta-adrenergic receptor blockers 3
Biliopancreatic diversion surgery 84
Birth
　asphyxia 159
　weight 89
Bleomycin 74, 75
Blindness 89
Blood
　glucose, self-monitored 164
　pressure 107, 108
Body mass index 82, 82*t*, 135, 147, 148
Brachial plexus injury 159
Breast 55
　cancer 32, 33, 55
　　survivors 38
　malignancy 32
Breastfeeding 16, 38

C

Calcium 84
Cancer 54, 72
　colorectal 55
　direct effect of 73
　effect of 73*fc*
　endometrial 46, 50, 51
　genes, hereditary 57
　hematological 65
　hereditary 54
　survivors 32, 46, 54, 61, 76, 79
Cardiac disease 107, 109, 111
Cardiovascular diseases 107
Cavernous nerve injury 74
Central nervous system tumors 73
Cervical carcinoma 64
Cesarean section 88
Chemotherapy 33, 36, 74
　risk of 74*fc*
Cholestasis, obstetric 134
Chorioamnionitis 125
Chorionic villus sampling 138
Cirrhosis 133, 139
Cisplatin 75

Clomiphene 122
   citrate 122
Colon 55
Comprehensive multidisciplinary fertility preservation 66
Computed tomography scan 47
Continuous glucose monitoring 164
Controlled ovarian
   hyperstimulation 14, 150
   stimulation 14, 35, 36, 49, 57, 65, 86, 108-110
Coronary artery disease 107
Corticosteroids 12
Cyclophosphamide therapy 93
Cyclosporine 12
Cystectomy 74
Cytomegalovirus 15

D

Dacarbazine 74
Deafness 89
Deep vein thrombosis 14
   pulmonary embolism of 99
Deoxyribonucleic acid 22, 55, 75, 132, 158
Diabetes mellitus 107, 157, 157b, 158b
   gestational 16, 85, 87-89, 125, 137, 160, 162
   type 1 157, 162
   type 2 157, 163
Diuretics 148
Dyslipidemia 148

E

Eclampsia 159
Egg freezing 63
Ejaculatory duct 74
Electrocardiography 109, 147
Embryo cryopreservation 135
Embryo freezing 62
Endometrium 118
Epigenetic dysregulation 158
Epilepsy 89
Erectile dysfunction 21, 22, 83, 120, 158
   treatment of 23
Estimated glomerular filtration rate 121
Estradiol 57
Etoposide 75

F

Failure to thrive 89
Female sexual function index score 118
Fertility 2, 32, 37, 46, 54, 61, 75, 76, 82, 92, 99, 107, 108f, 109, 115, 116fc, 131, 146, 157

   female 85t, 116
   issues 131
   male 20, 24, 72-74, 74fc, 85t, 119
   preservation 33, 35, 46, 51, 57, 61, 62fc, 66
      methods of 76, 76fc
   rates 132
Fetal
   anomalies 88
   blood sampling 138
   growth restriction 12, 88, 93, 149
Folate 84
Follicle-stimulating hormone 3, 13, 23, 33, 101, 116, 123
Folliculogenesis 33
Frozen embryo transfer 150

G

Gamete 135
   preparation 135
Gamma-glutamyltransferase 136
Gastric band
   erosion 89
   slipping of 89
Gastrointestinal disorder 94
Gestational age
   large for 164
   small for 14, 85
Glomerular filtration rate 119
Glucose monitoring timing 164
Glycemic targets 160
Gonadal dysfunction 3
Gonadal shielding 64
Gonadotoxicity, risk of 61
Gonadotropin-releasing hormone 13, 20, 61, 116, 117
   agonist 62, 86, 123
   analogs 63
   antagonists 14, 124
Graft
   function 6
   rejection 15
Growth retardation 89

H

Hashimoto's thyroiditis 157
Heart disease 108f
   congenital 108, 109
   cyanotic 109
Hemangioma, hepatic 137
Hematological malignancies 61, 66
Hemolysis, elevated liver enzymes, and low platelet syndrome 14, 149

Hemorrhage
  antepartum 138
  cerebral 89
  postpartum 87, 138, 149
Hepatitis 137
  A 138
    virus 132, 134
  autoimmune 131, 134, 137
  B 132, 137, 138
    infection 135
    surface antigen 134
    virus 131, 132, 134
  C 132, 137, 138
    virus 24, 131, 132, 134
  D 132, 138
    virus 132
  E 138
    virus 132
  type 138
  viral 132, 133
  viruses 138t
Hereditary cancer syndrome, management strategies for 58
Heterotopic transplantation 64
Heterozygote 102
Hodgkin's disease 74, 75
Hodgkin's lymphoma 61, 72
Homozygote 102
Hormonal disturbances 3
  treatment of 23
Hormone therapy 34
Human chorionic gonadotropin 73, 86, 123
Human immunodeficiency virus 15, 137, 138
Human menopausal gonadotropin 101
Hydroxychloroquine 94
Hyperandrogenism 157
Hyperbilirubinemia 159
Hyperhomocysteinemia 103
Hyperplasia, endometrial 46
Hypertension 15, 93, 107, 146, 147, 147b, 149
  chronic 146, 151, 152b
  portal 140
  pregnancy-induced 85, 125
Hypertensive disorders 146, 148, 151
Hypocalcemia 159
Hypoglycemia 159
  management of 164
Hypogonadism 158
Hypomagnesemia 159
Hypothalamic-pituitary-gonadal axis 20, 73, 75, 83

Hypothalamic-pituitary-ovarian
  axis 85
  dysfunction 117f
Hypothyroidism 162

I

Immunosuppressants 11
Immunosuppression 5
In vitro fertilization 2, 10, 13, 35, 48, 56, 63, 78, 99, 100, 102t, 110, 134, 135t, 146, 161
  complications of 14
In vitro maturation 36, 62, 65
Infections 15
  congenital 16
Infertility 1, 25, 99
  etiopathogenesis of 2
  male 111
  malignancy-induced 73
Insulin use 163
Intensive care unit 5, 149
Intracytoplasmic sperm injection 56, 78, 134, 150
Intrauterine death 159
Intrauterine insemination 48
Intussusception 89
Iron 84
Irritable bowel syndrome 92, 94

K

Kidney
  disease
    chronic 20, 22, 23, 115, 117f, 121
    end-stage 116
  dysfunction 116, 117
  injury, acute 124, 125

L

Leukemia 61, 72, 73
  acute lymphocytic 61
  acute myeloid 61
  lymphoblastic 78
Leukopenia 95
Levonorgestrel intrauterine device 50
Leydig cells 119
Live birth rate 13, 33, 50
Liver 136f
  disease 24, 25, 131, 134
    alcoholic 133, 139
    chronic 20, 131, 141
    influence of 24

disorders 131
dysfunction 134
function 136*f*
physiology 136
transplant 134, 141
Low anterior colonic resection 74
Lower segment cesarean section 87
Low-molecular weight heparin 14, 103
Luteinizing hormone 3, 21, 33, 116, 117, 123
Lymphoma 61, 73
Lynch syndrome 55

M

Macrosomia 87, 159
    fetal 164
Magnetic resonance imaging 47, 108, 134
Malignant cells, transmission of 78
Malnutrition 88
Marfan syndrome 108
Mean arterial pressure 148
Menarche, late 157
Menopause, premature 157
Menstrual abnormalities 157
Menstrual cycle 117
Metformin 51, 161, 164
Microsurgical epididymal sperm aspiration 77
Miscarriage 87, 159
    first-trimester 124
Mycophenolate mofetil 11
Myocardial infarction 149

N

Neoadjuvant chemotherapy 39
Neonatal intensive care unit 90
Neural tube defects 89
Nonalcoholic fatty liver disease 131, 134, 136
Non-Hodgkin's lymphoma 61
Nuchal translucency 86
Nutritional deficiencies 88

O

Obesity 82, 83, 86
    effect of 82
    juvenile 88
Oncofertility 49, 61
Oncotherapy 79, 80
Oocyte
    cryopreservation 35

development 33
in vitro maturation of 65
pickup 161
Oogenesis 33
Oophoropexy 64
Operative vaginal delivery 87
Oral contraceptive pills 85
Oral glucose tolerance test 87
Oral medroxy progesterone acetate 50
Oral megestrol acetate 50
Orthotopic transplantation 64
Ovarian hyperstimulation syndrome 13, 57, 100, 102, 103, 107, 115, 124, 134, 149, 161
Ovarian reserve 118
Ovarian stimulation 149
Ovarian tissue
    cryopreservation 35, 49, 64
    freezing 64
    transplantation 64

P

Pelvic sarcoma 64
Percutaneous epididymal sperm aspiration 77
Perinatal death 89
Peritonitis, life-threatening 89
Phosphodiesterase-5 inhibitors 23
Placental abruption 149
Polycystic ovarian syndrome 46, 85, 103, 107, 132, 157, 161
Polycythemia 159
Postbariatric surgery 82, 86
Preconceptional counseling 11, 26, 55, 83, 94, 108, 120, 147, 147*b*, 158
Preeclampsia 87, 159
Pregnancy 6, 37, 38, 51, 85, 100, 135, 136
    ectopic 124
    effect of 4, 121, 163
    hypertensive disorders of 148
    multiple 125
    outcome 38, 50
    postbariatric surgery, care of 88
    rate 48
Preimplantation genetic testing 56
Premature ovarian insufficiency 61
Prepregnancy counseling 133, 133*t*
Preterm birth 89, 134
Progesterone 51
Prolactin 21
Propranolol 148
Prostatectomy 74
Prothrombin time 136

R

Radiation therapy 75
Radiotherapy 35
　effect of 75*fc*
Randomized controlled trials 75
Rapamycin, mammalian target of 134
Recurrent pregnancy loss 83
Renal disease 115
　chronic 115
　effect of 116, 116*fc*, 119
　end-stage 2, 20, 21, 115
Renal insufficiency 149
Renal replacement therapy 122
Renal transplantation 2, 22
　effect of 22
Reproductive period, shortening of 157
Respiratory distress syndrome 159
Retroperitoneal lymph node dissection 74
Ribonucleic acid 24, 134
Rivaroxaban 100
Roux-en-Y gastric bypass 84

S

Selective estrogen receptor modulator 122
Semen
　analysis 119
　freezing 77
Seminal vesicle 74
Severe preeclampsia management 153*fc*
Sex hormone 85
　binding globulin 85, 131
Sexual dysfunction 23, 25, 85, 157
Sexual function 24, 85, 118, 120
Shoulder dystocia 159
Single-embryo transfer 14
Sleeve gastrectomy 84
Small bowel obstruction 89
Solid organ transplants 20
Sperm 77
　parameters 21
Spermatogenesis 72, 158
　impairment of 158
Spermatogenic function, poor recovery
　　of 119
Spermatogonial stem cells 66, 78
Spermatozoa, cryopreservation of 77
Steatohepatitis, nonalcoholic 131
Stem cells reproductive technologies 65
Stillbirth 159
Stroke 149
Subfertility, male 158
Surgery, effect of 74
Systemic lupus erythematosus 92

T

Tacrolimus 12
Tamoxifen 51
Testicular germ cell tumors 72
Testicular sperm
　aspiration 77
　extraction 66, 77
Testicular tissue 66
　cryopreservation 78
Testosterone
　concentration 158
　replacement therapy 25
Thiazides 3
Thrombocytopenia 95
Thromboembolic episode, risk
　　period of 100
Thromboembolism 103
　risk of 100
Thromboprophylaxis 99, 102*t*
　action plan for 103*t*
Thyroid stimulating hormone 162
Total body irradiation 61
Toxoplasma 15
Tracheoesophageal fistula 159
Transvaginal sonography 86
Transvaginal ultrasound 48
Turner syndrome 108

U

Ulcer, gastric 89
Ultrasonography 14, 87, 162

V

Vaginal birth after cesarean 87
Vaginal carcinoma 64
Vas deferens 74
Venous thromboembolism 87, 99, 102,
　　103, 110, 125
Vertebral defects 159
Vinblastine 74
Vitamin
　B12 84
　D 84
　　deficiency 15
　K antagonists 100
Volvulus 89

W

Weight gain, gestational 89

www.ingramcontent.com/pod-product-compliance
Ingram Content Group UK Ltd.
Pitfield, Milton Keynes, MK11 3LW, UK
UKHW052202140425
457402UK00003B/17